Trevor Sorbie: The Bridal Hair Book

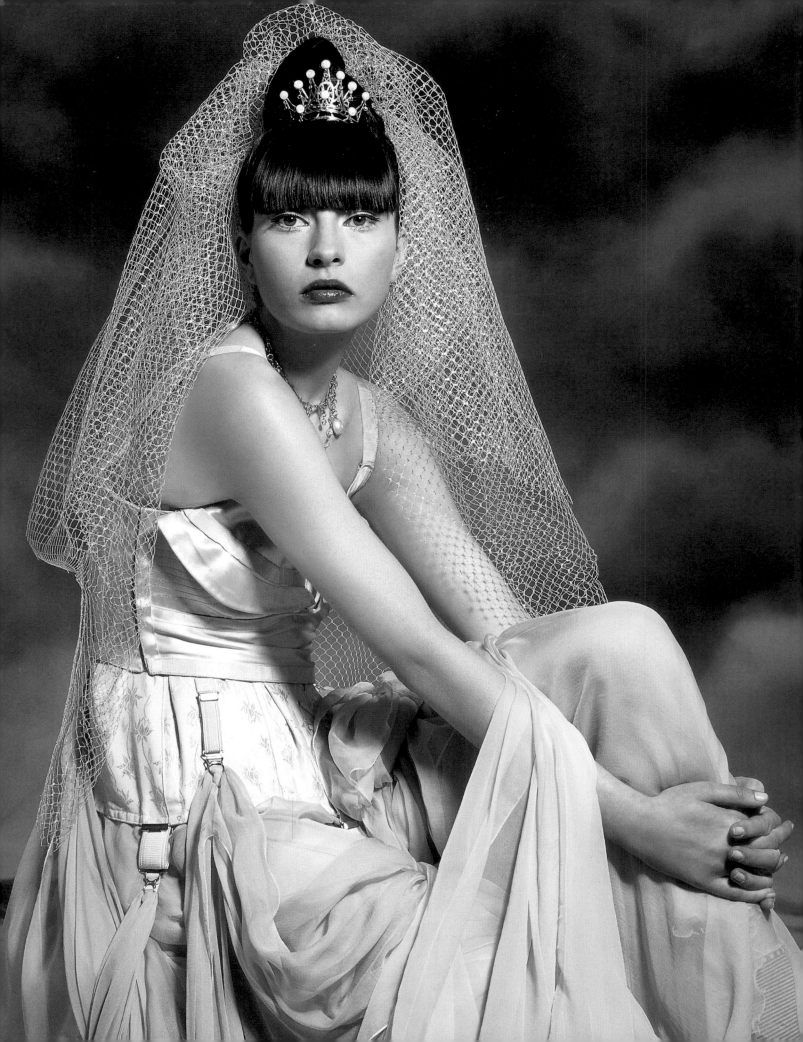

TREVOR SORBIE AND JACKI WADESON

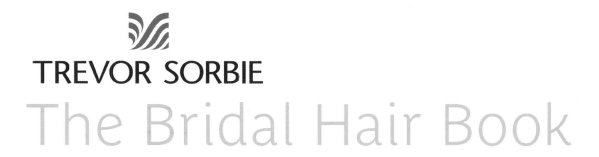

TREVOR SORBIE
The Bridal Hair Book

24 step-by-step techniques

Photography: Barry Cook

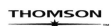 THOMSON™   habia   City& Guilds

Australia • Canada • Mexico • Singapore • Spain • United Kingdom • United States

With special thanks to Daniel Caceres who was responsible for interpreting my ideas and translating them into these stunning step-by-steps. Well done Daniel.

TREVOR SORBIE

THOMSON

Trevor Sorbie – The Bridal Hair Book

Copyright © 2006 Thomson Learning

The Thomson logo is a registered trademark used herein under licence.

For more information, contact Thomson Learning, High Holborn House, 50–51 Bedford Row, London WC1R 4LR or visit us on the World Wide Web at: http://www.thomsonlearning.co.uk

British Library Cataloguing-in-Publication Data
A catalogue record for this book is available from the British Library

ISBN-13: 978-1-84480-324-8
ISBN-10: 1-84480-324-4

Published in 2006 by Thomson Learning

Designed and typeset by LewisHallam
Printed in Italy by Canale

Contents

ACKNOWLEDGEMENTS   6

INTRODUCTION   9

BOHO CHIC

1   French Pleat   12
2   Fishtail   18
3   Top Knot   24
4   Rope Braid   30

CLASSIC

5   Twisted Ponytails   38
6   50s Bouffant   44
7   Audrey Hepburn   50
8   Short to Long   54
9   Finger Waves   60
10   Top Twist   64

GLAMOROUS

11   Bridget Bardot   70
12   Coloured Wefts   76
13   Frizz   82
14   Twiglets   88

ROMANTIC

15   Spiral Curls   94
16   Scarlett O'Hara   100
17   Dreadlocks   106
18   Coils   112
19   Twist 'n' Dry   118

TECHNIQUES

Basic Blow Drying   126
Herringbone Braid   128
Marcel Wave   130
Root Curl Tonging   132
Spiral Tonging   134

MARKETING

Reaping rewards from your bridal service   138

CREDITS

Clothes and accessories   142

Acknowledgements

HAIR: Trevor Sorbie and Daniel Caceres

Assisted by the Trevor Sorbie Artistic Team

PRODUCTS: Trevor Sorbie Professional

HAIRPIECES: Trendco and Hairaisers

CLOTHES STYLING: Wendy Elsmore, Kathy Burch (Mrs O),
David O'Brian

MAKE-UP: Madeline Hale and Ailton Americo

PHOTOGRAPHY: Barry Cook

PHOTOGRAPHY ASSISTANT: Charley Crittenden

EDITOR: Jacki Wadeson

www.trevorsorbie.com

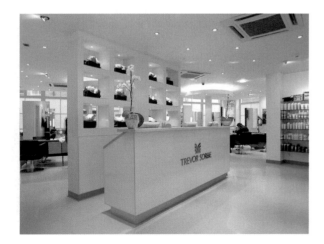

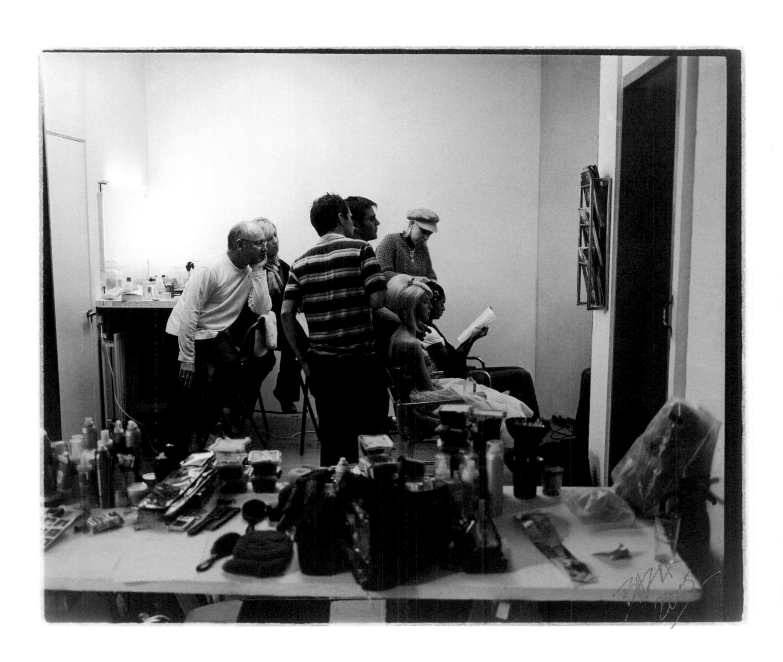

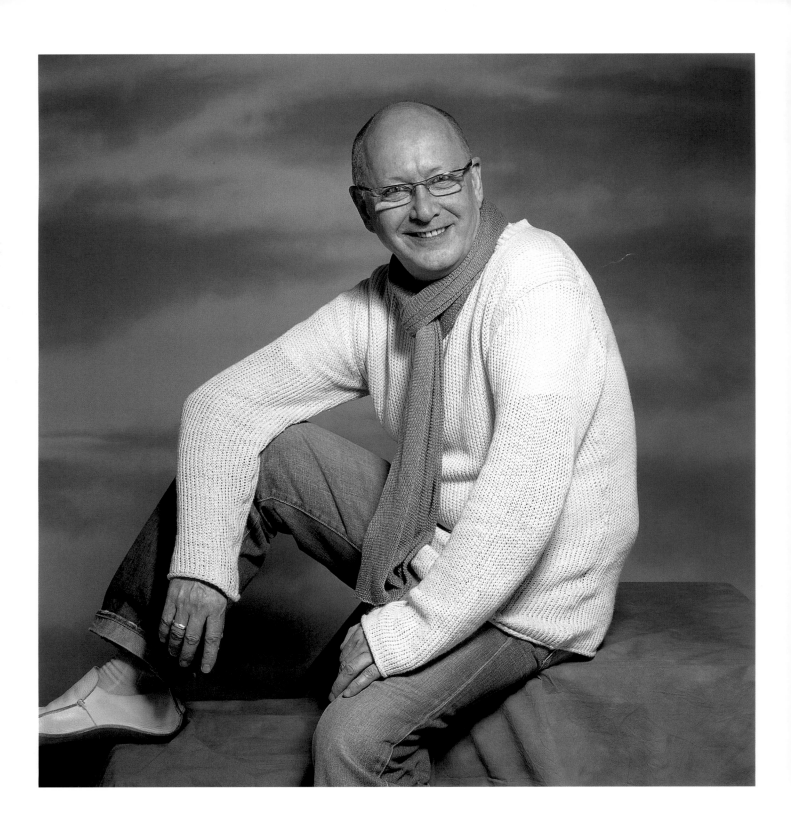

Introduction

Welcome to my interpretation of one of our most traditional rituals – the wedding.

Unlike many of my clients, my feelings on 'dressed' hair were not love at first sight! At the beginning of my career at a small suburban salon, Henri's in Loughton, Essex, where Saturday was always 'Wedding Day', I dreaded seeing an appointment for a 'hair up' in the client book, preferring instead to get creative with the clippers.

When my first bride appeared I panicked, faced with a fabulous head of long, thick, red hair and a request for ringlets I just couldn't deliver. Two hours under the dryer and one complaint later left both of us red-faced! My confidence shot, I vowed to myself it wouldn't happen again and decided to teach myself the demands of the wedding 'hair do'.

Happily I turned my weakness into a strength, and now after a great deal of learning and practice (and more practice), I can confidently say I enjoy creating beautiful styles which guarantee happy brides.

Wedding or Special Occasion hair is a service that fulfils your client's needs and gives you an opportunity to celebrate with them. This book can be your learning tool and guide. As your clients seek to personalise their wedding day to set it apart from the traditional, this book can provide some much needed inspiration.

My step-by-steps will create fresh looks to delight the modern-day bride and take the fear factor out of the challenge for you. I hope you enjoy reading and trying the styles as much as I enjoyed putting the ideas and book together.

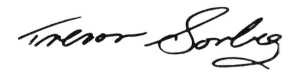

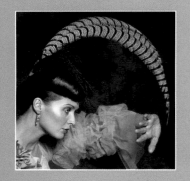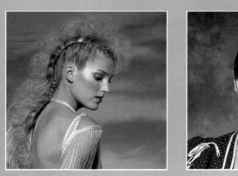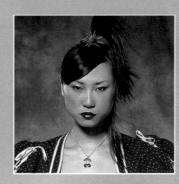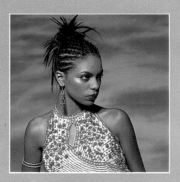

BOHO CHIC

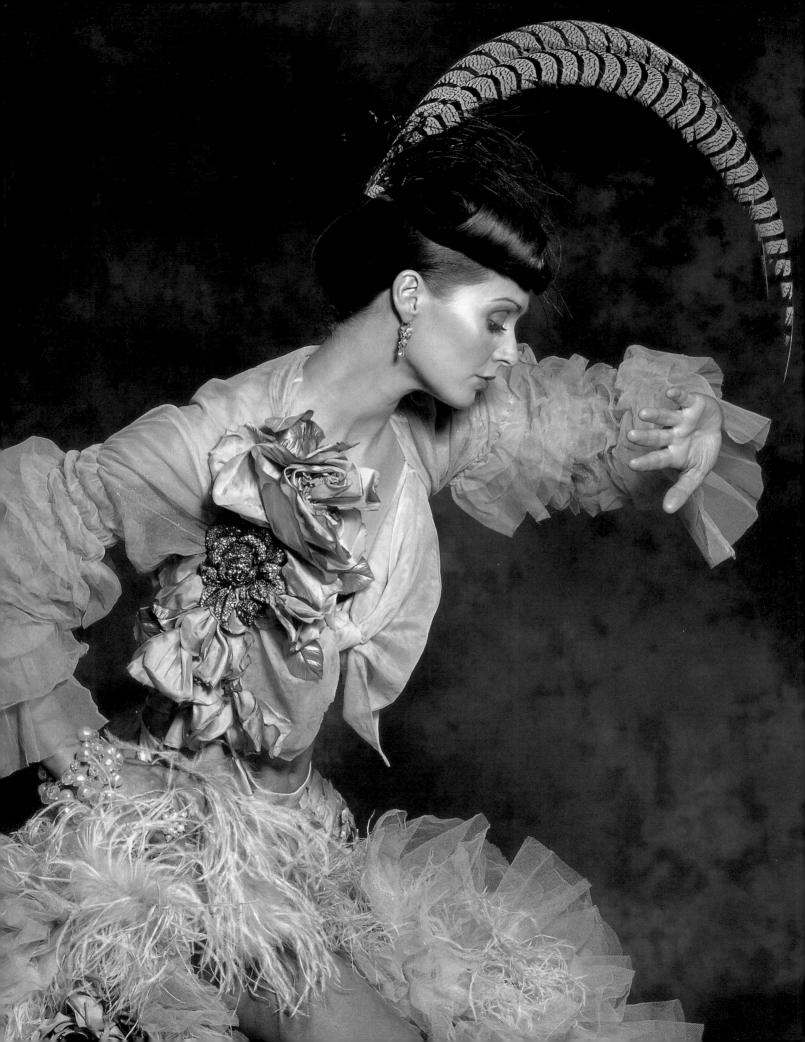

1 French Pleat

'A classic chignon is made
extraordinary by the addition of
this dramatic feather accessory.'

TREVOR SORBIE

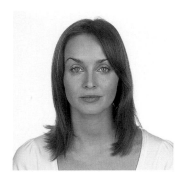

1 Before.

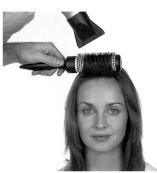

2 Blow dry first section of hair using a ceramic round bristle brush.

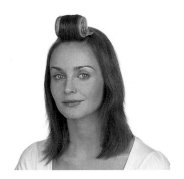

3 Now wind this section onto a self-fixing roller.

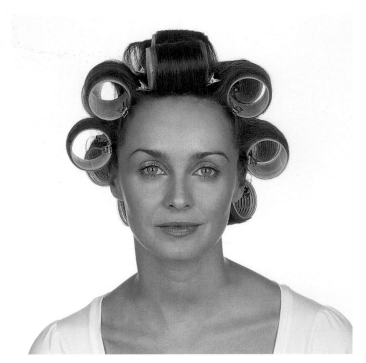

4 Shows completed pli.

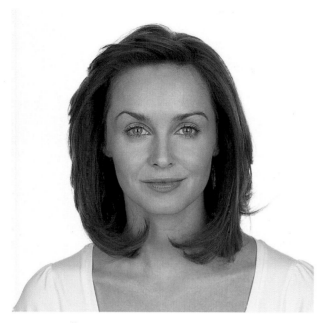

5 Remove rollers.

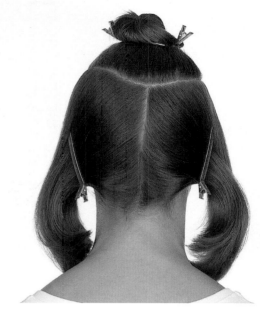

6 Section hair as shown.

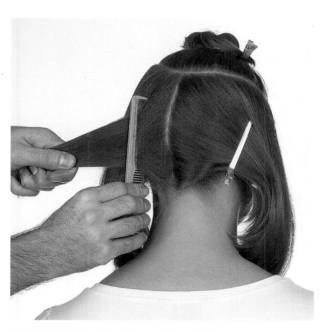

7 Backcomb one side of back sectioned hair.

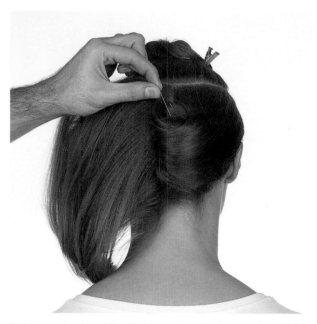

8 Backcomb other side of back sectioned hair, smooth and fold over into a pleat at centre back. Secure with pins.

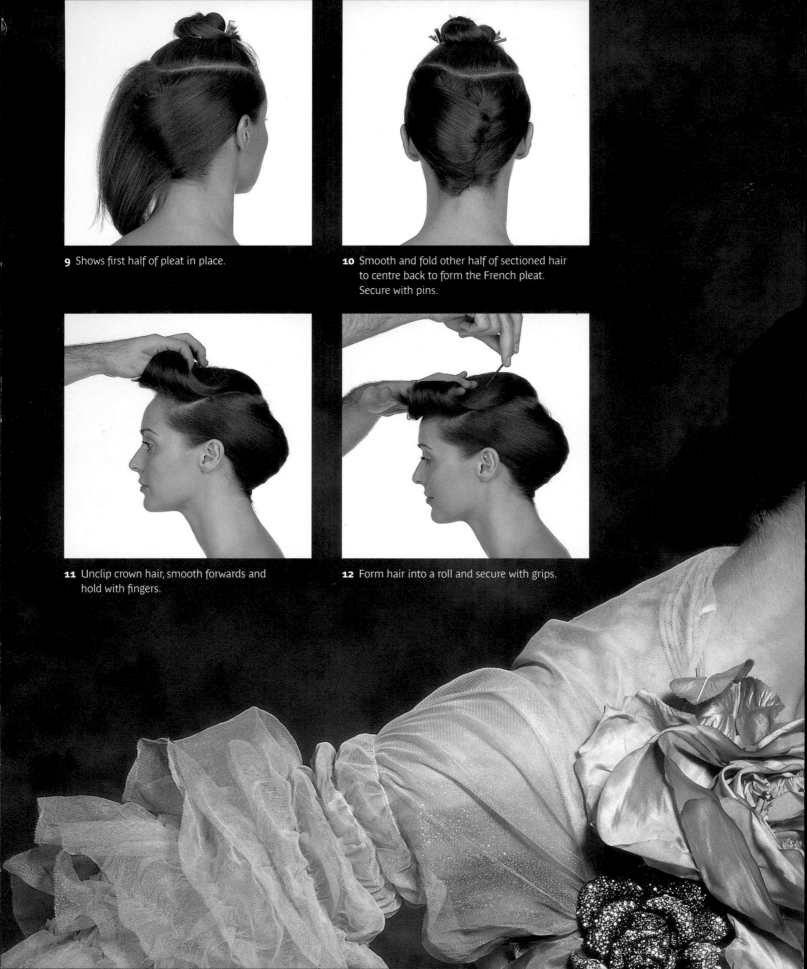

9 Shows first half of pleat in place.

10 Smooth and fold other half of sectioned hair to centre back to form the French pleat. Secure with pins.

11 Unclip crown hair, smooth forwards and hold with fingers.

12 Form hair into a roll and secure with grips.

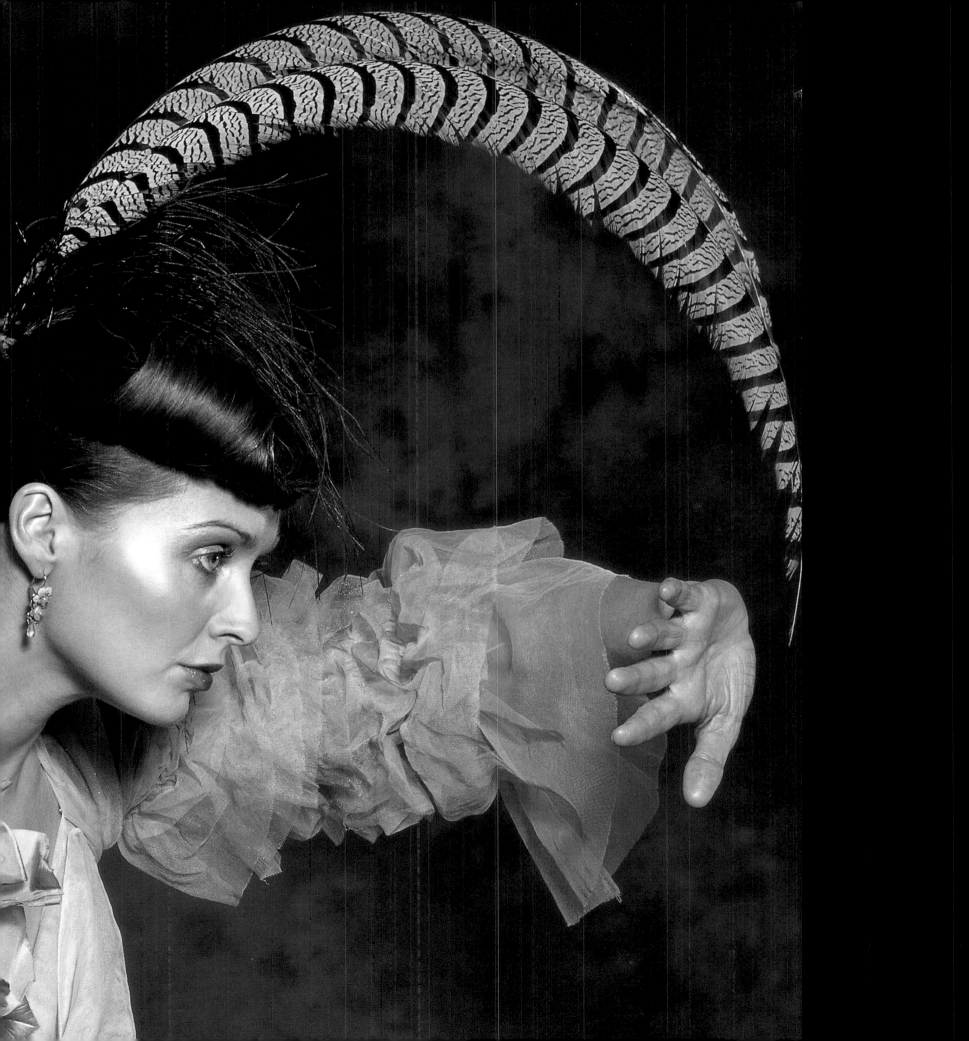

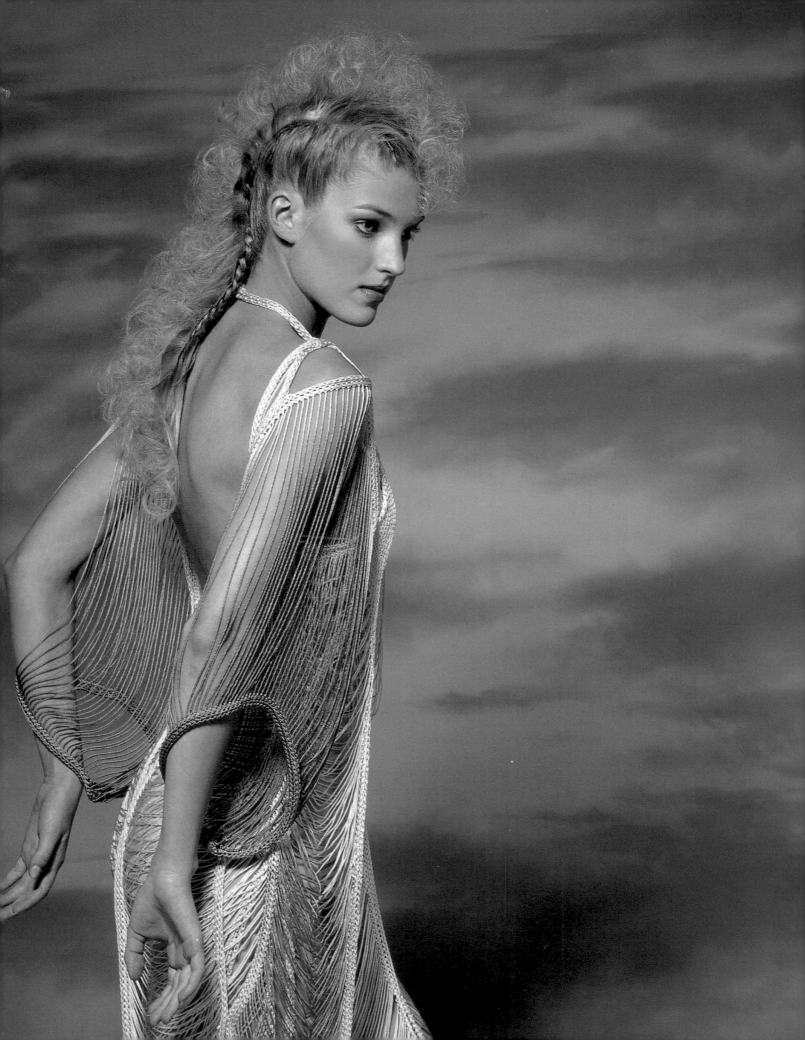

2 Fishtail

'The clever use of a simple weft, which has been curled then split into two, gives this most unusual yet dramatic result, not for the faint hearted.'

TREVOR SORBIE

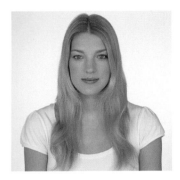

1 Before.

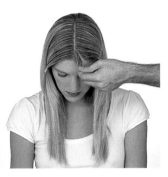

2 Part hair from centre front to centre back at nape. Now take a small diagonal section at front.

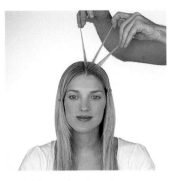

3 Divide section into three equal pieces.

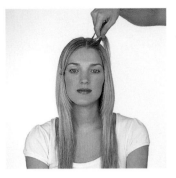

4 Work a basic 3-strand plait for 1.25 cm.

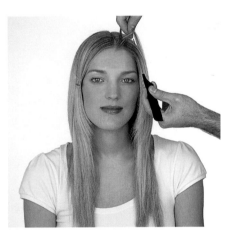

5 Use a tail comb to take a fine section from hairline and join to outer strand of already plaited hair.

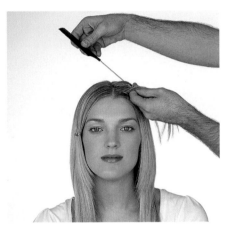

6 Take another section from side of centre parting as before and incorporate into plait. Continue working in same manner adding in first a fine section then a larger section to plait.

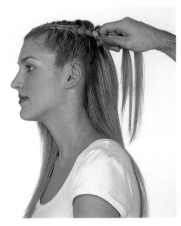

7 Shows plait forming at one side. Continue plaiting, in same manner, until you reach ends of hair and secure with a band.

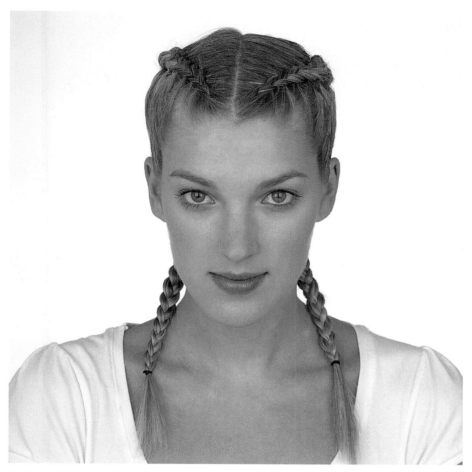

8 Shows plaiting completed.

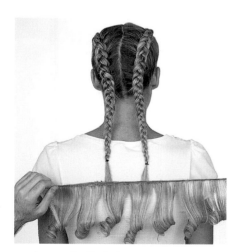

9 Take a weft of hair that has been tonged to form curls.

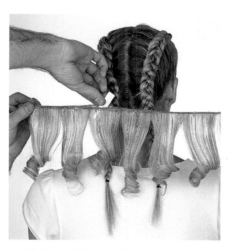

10 Divide weft into two by running a razor along top edge.

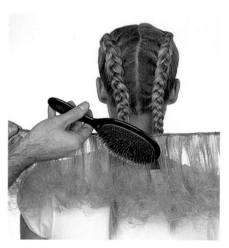

11 Back brush weft to tousle curls.

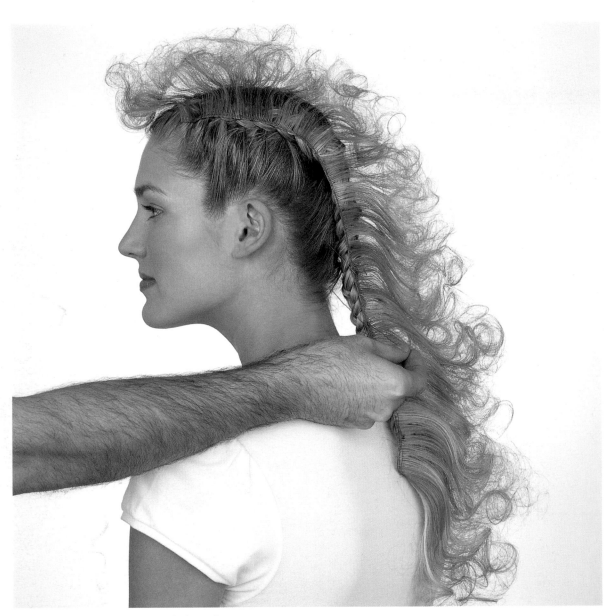

12 Pin weft in place over previously formed
plaits at each side of head.

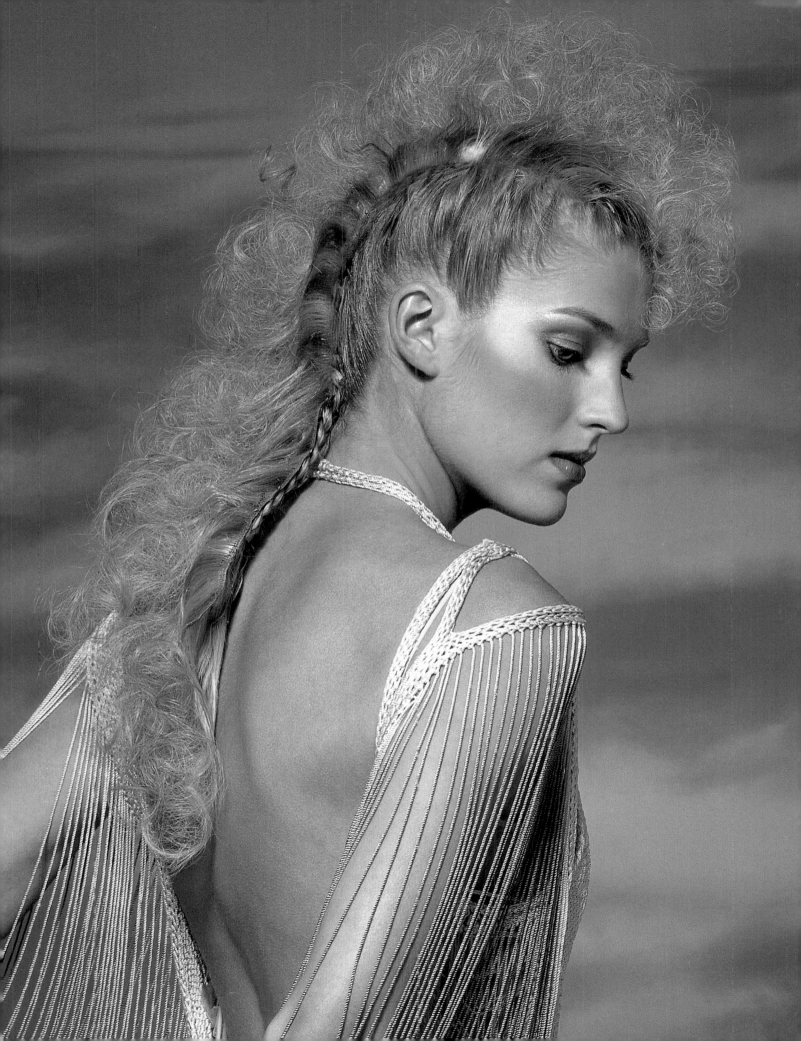

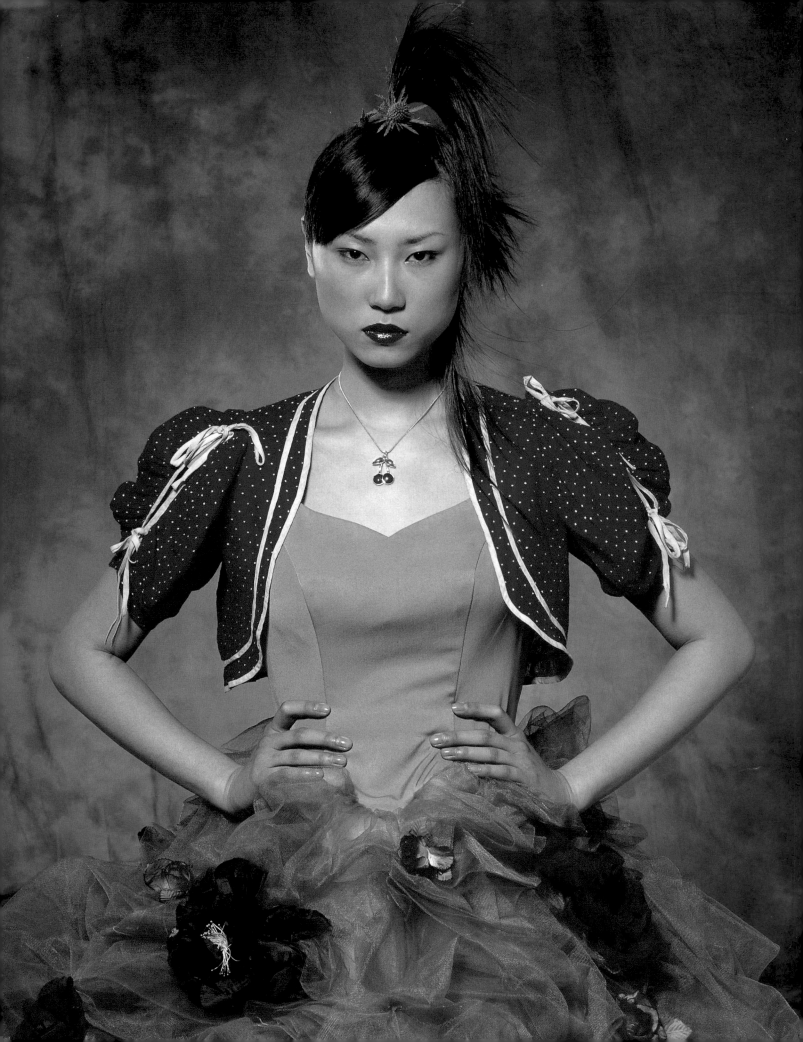

3 Top Knot

'The ultimate in simplicity is created by using two ponytails which utilize the quality of Asian hair to give a soft, spiky result.'

TREVOR SORBIE

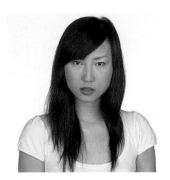 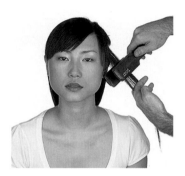 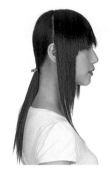

1 Before.

2 Straighten hair, one section at a time, using smoothing irons.

3 Divide off front hair and clip back hair as shown.

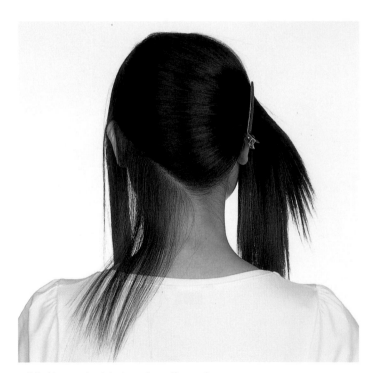

4 Working on back hair make a diagonal parting from ear to middle of nape.

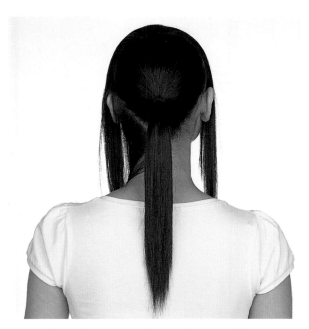

5 Smooth remaining back hair into a low ponytail, secure with a band.

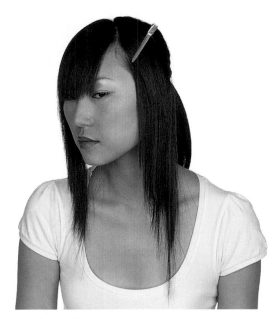

6 Return to front hair.

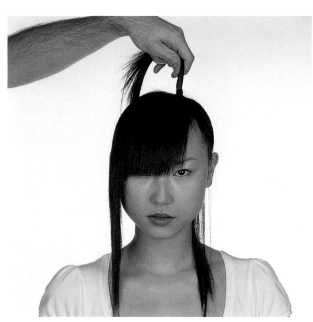

7 Smooth one side up to crown and secure in a ponytail with a band.

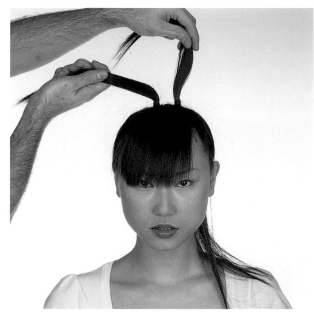

8 Do the same with other side of hair, then secure both ponytails together with another band.

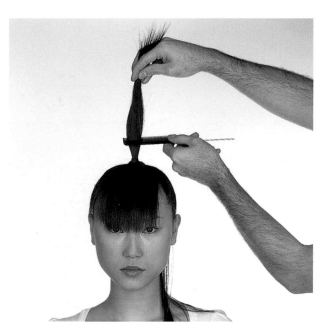

9 Backcomb base of ponytail so hair forms a tuft. Mist with hairspray.

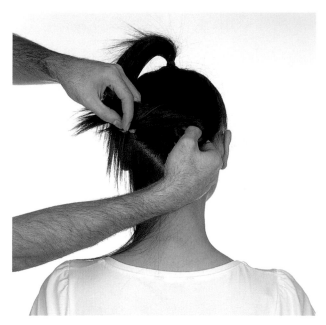

10 Twist back ponytail into a coil, allowing ends to splay out, then secure with grips. Allow other remaining section to fall free. Comb fringe to side.

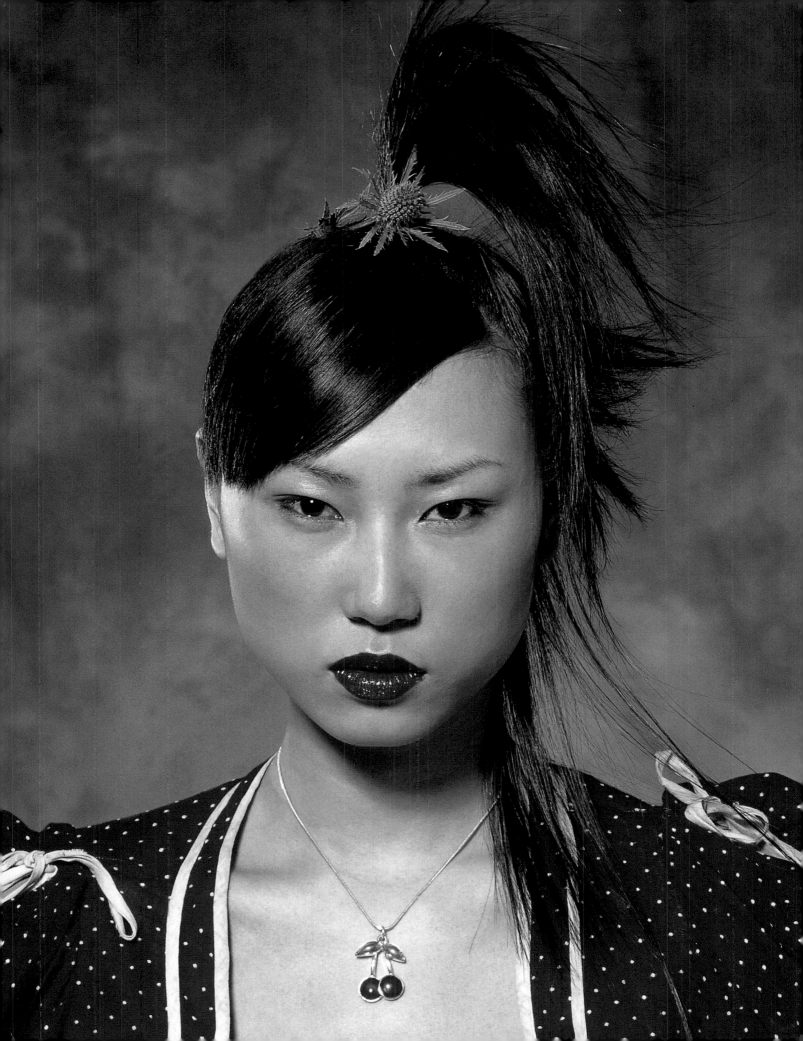

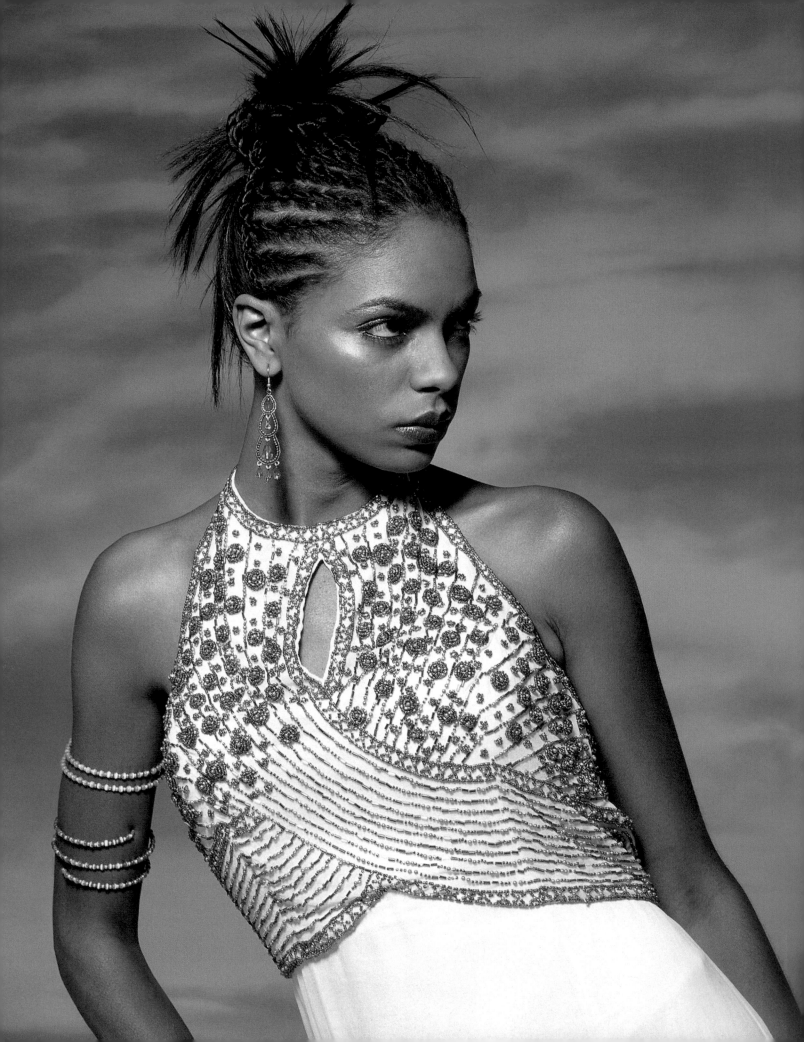

4 Rope Braid

'Using a braiding technique and leaving the ends out, we have created a look that reminds me of what an ethnic princess would look like.'

TREVOR SORBIE

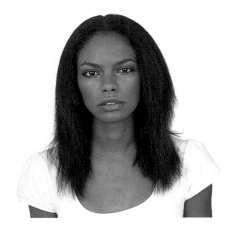

1 Before.

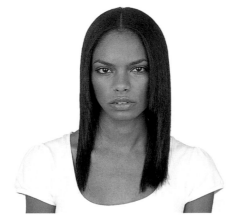

2 Hair is straightened, one section at a time, using smoothing irons.

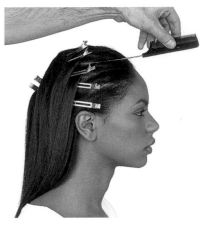

3 Comb hair straight back from hairline and use a tail comb to divide hair into working sections. Clip each section.

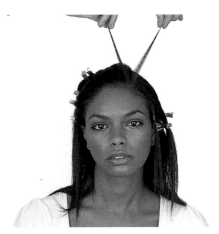

4 Take a half an inch square from first section you will be working on, then divide this into two equal sections.

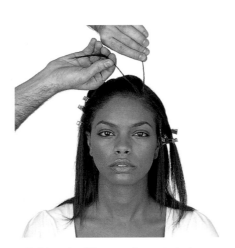

5 Twist each of these sections clockwise.

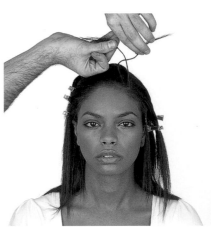

6 Cross over these sections anti-clockwise, i.e. right over left.

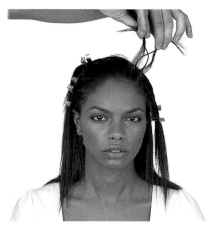 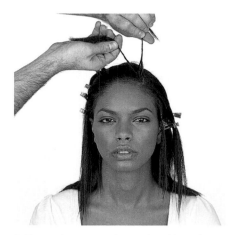

7 Take next half an inch square from your working section and again divide into two equal sections. Join each new section to each previously twisted section as before.

8 Shows the new sections twisted into the previously worked sections.

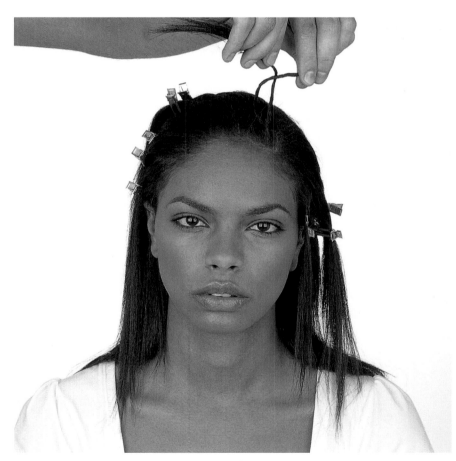

9 Cross over anti-clockwise again as before. Continue plaiting in same way to ends of each section.

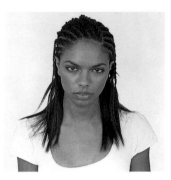

10 Shows plaits completed.

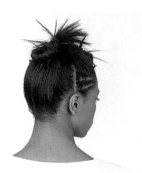

11 Smooth back hair up to centre back, twist and knot allowing ends to splay out. Grip in place.

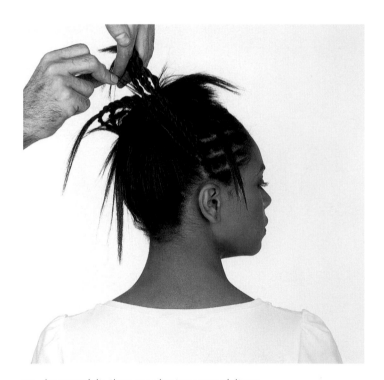

12 Arrange plaits then use pins to secure plaits on top of head.

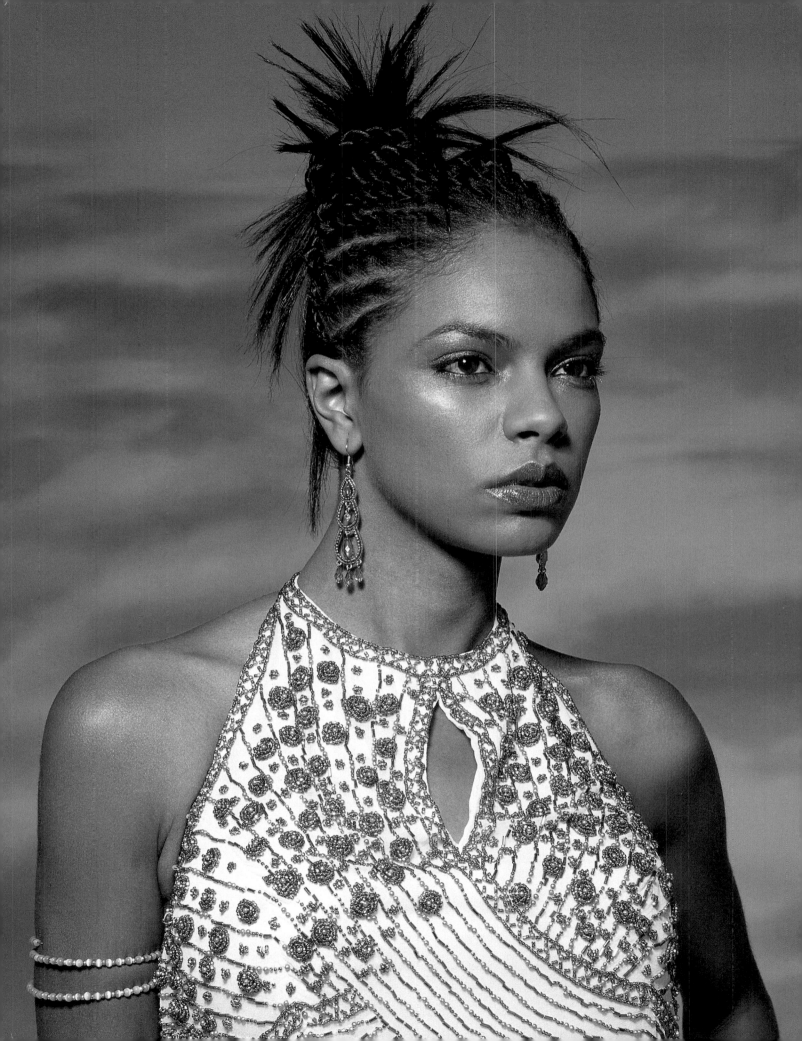

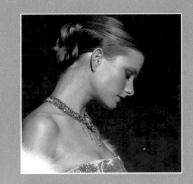

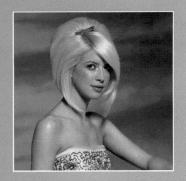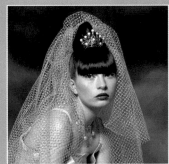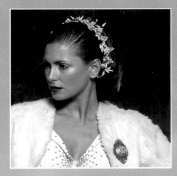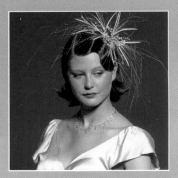

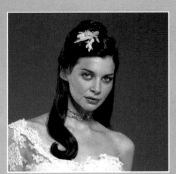

CLASSIC

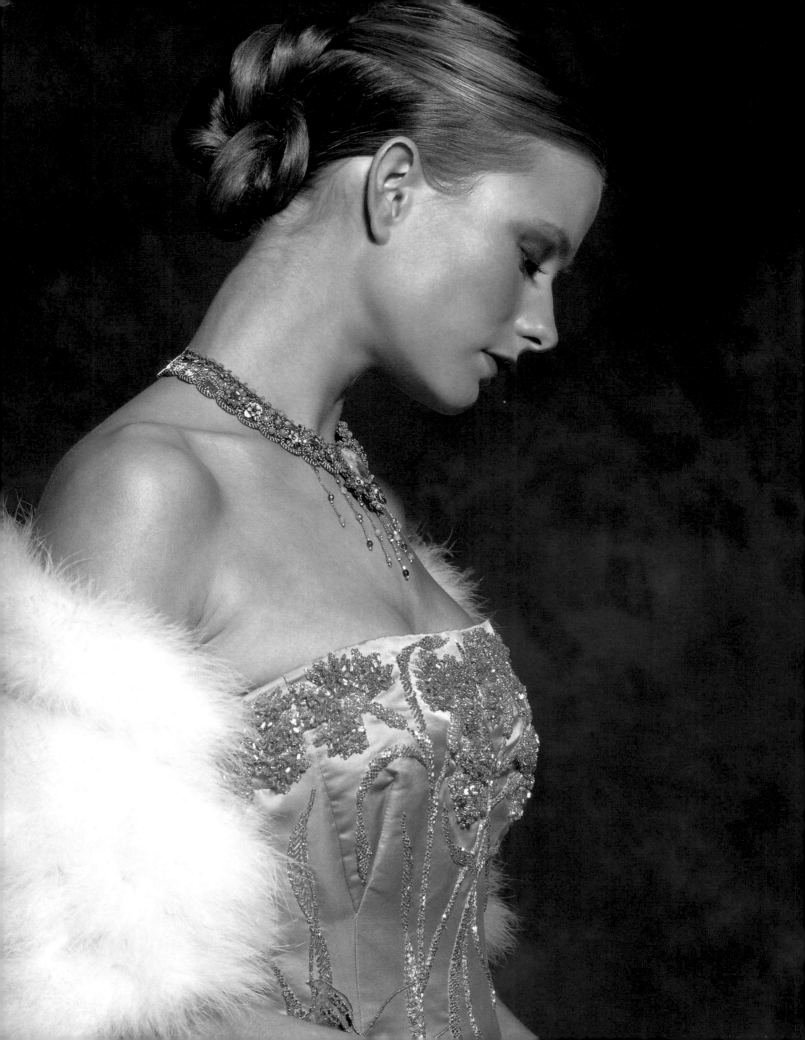

5 Twisted Ponytails

'By using invisible hair nets, we have taken the difficulty out of doing a classic French chignon.'

TREVOR SORBIE

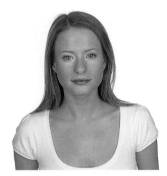

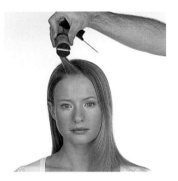

1 Before.

2 From a side parting, section hair and set on heated rollers.

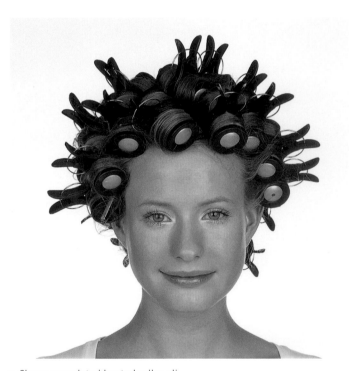

3 Shows completed heated roller pli.

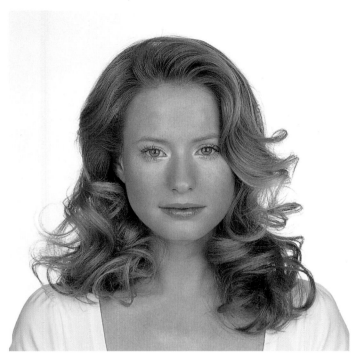

4 Remove rollers and allow hair to fall free.

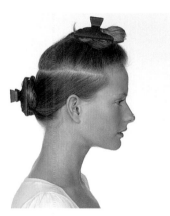

5 Section hair and clip as shown.

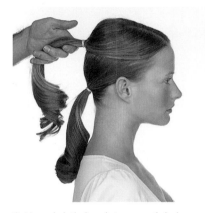

6 Use a bristle brush to smooth hair into upper and lower ponytails, then secure with bands.

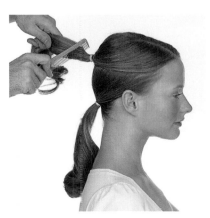

7 Backcomb each ponytail.

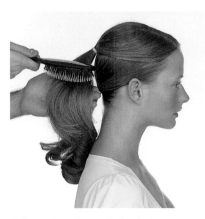

8 Smooth each ponytail using a bristle brush.

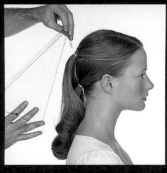

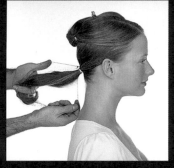

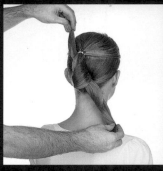

9 Take a fine hairnet and spread out between fingers.

10 Encase lower ponytail in fine hairnet and secure by gripping one edge to band. Repeat for upper ponytail.

11 Knot ponytails together. This is easy now the hair is enclosed in the nets.

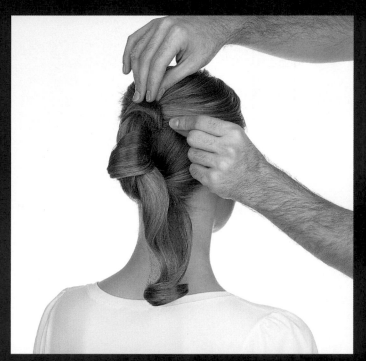

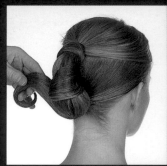

13 Loop round tail of other ponytail, secure with grips.

12 Pin round ends of lower ponytail as shown, secure with grips.

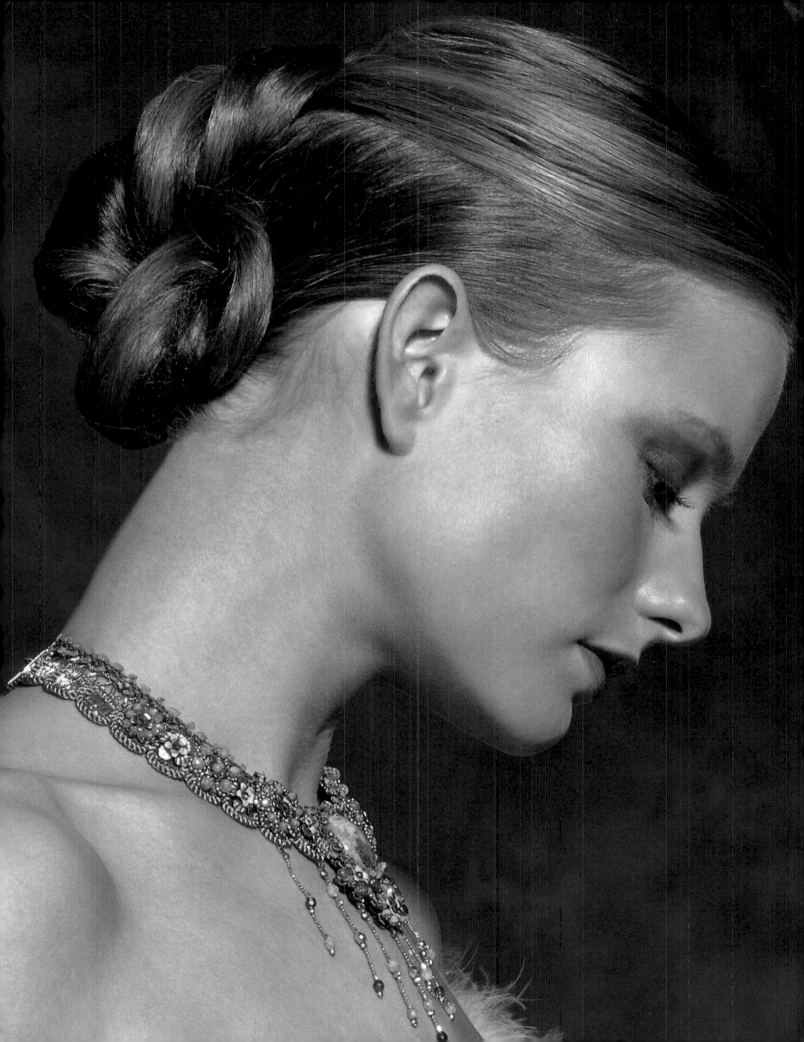

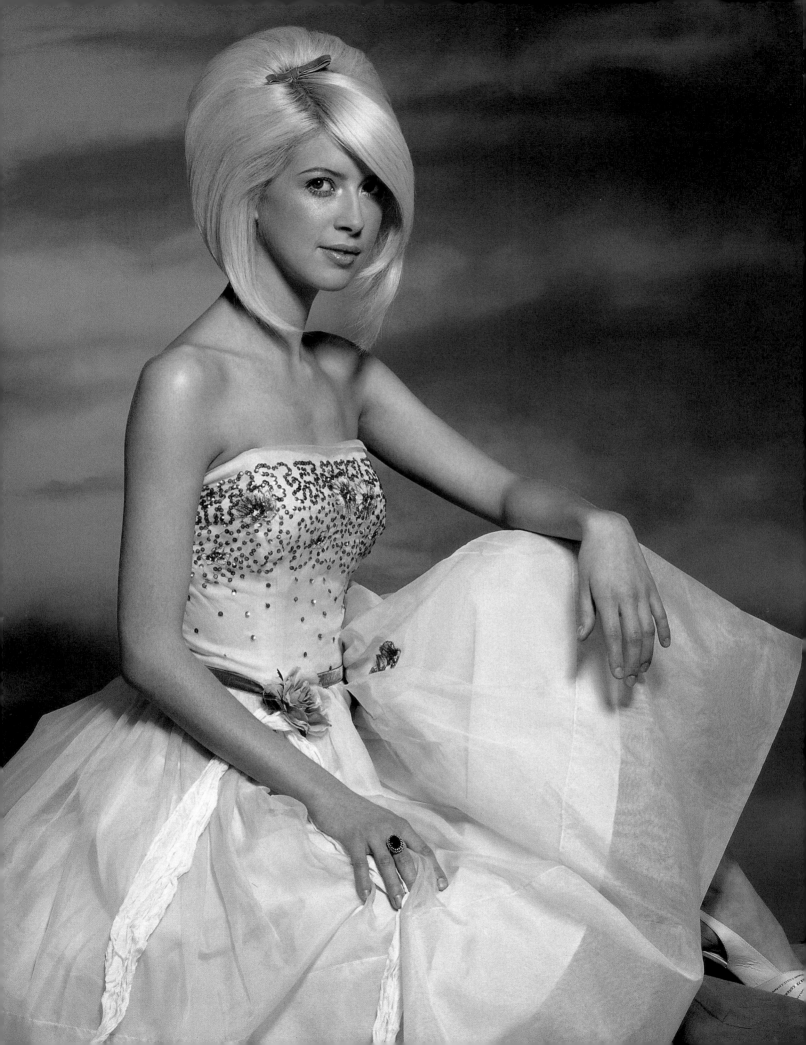

6 50s Bouffant

'Using a layered bob as a base, we added a 50s twist by the use of backbrushing to give a modern take on the bouffant.'

TREVOR SORBIE

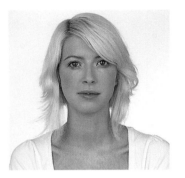

1 Before.

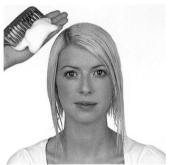

2 Apply a generous amount of mousse to damp hair.

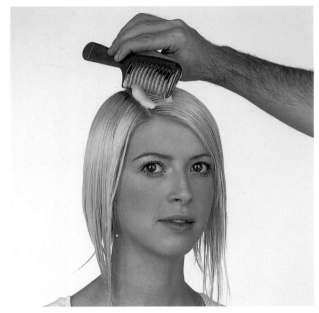

3 Starting at parting, use a wide tooth comb to distribute mousse through hair.

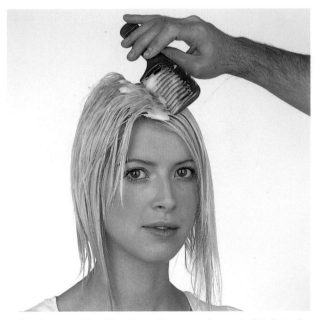

4 Continue working like this until mousse is evenly distributed.

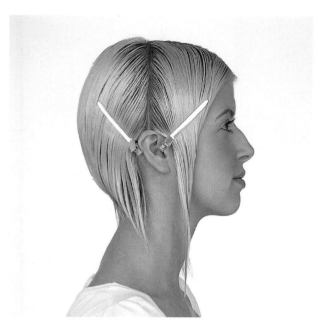

5 Section hair as shown.

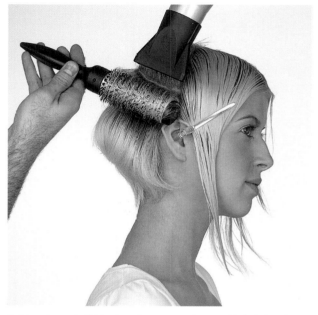

6 Blow dry to build body using a ceramic round bristle brush, pointing dryer down the hair shaft to maximise shine.

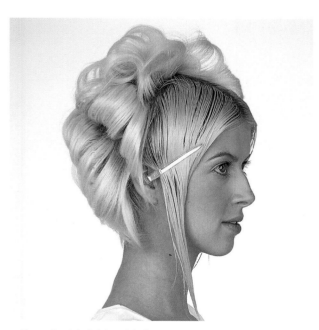

7 Shows back hair blow dried.

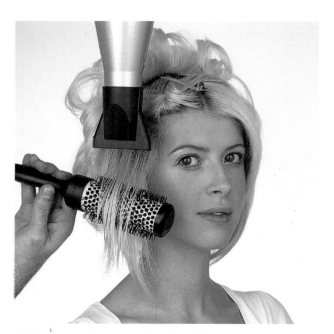

8 Blow dry front hair smooth and straight using a ceramic round bristle brush.

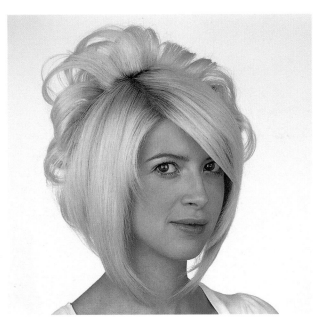

9 Shows completed blow dry.

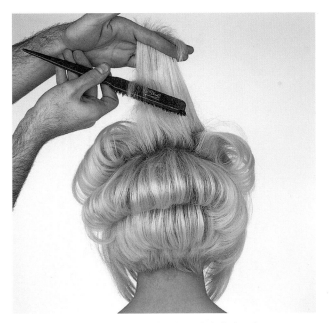

10 Backcomb hair then smooth using a bristle brush.

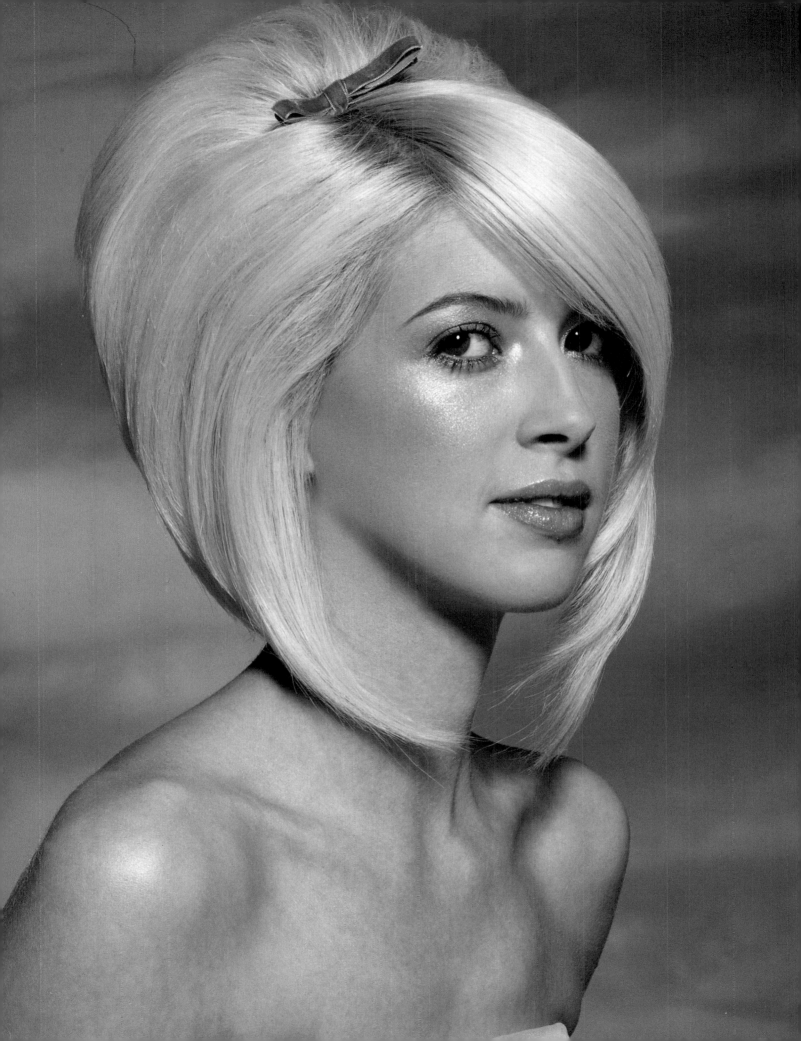

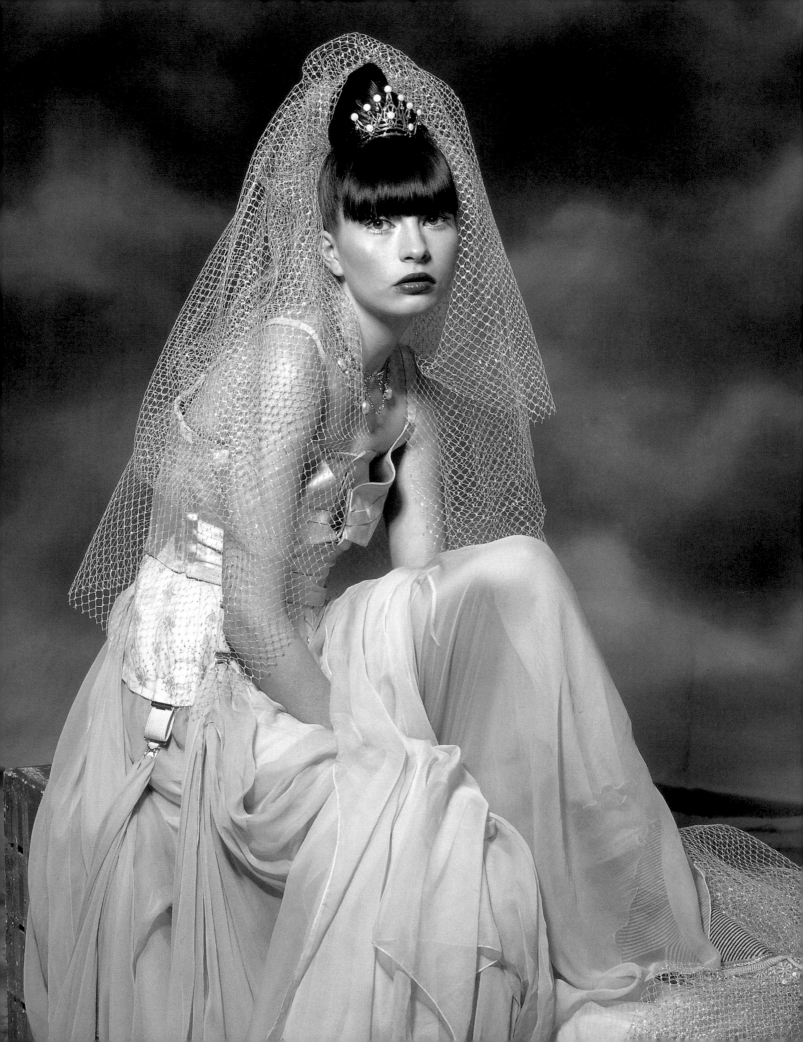

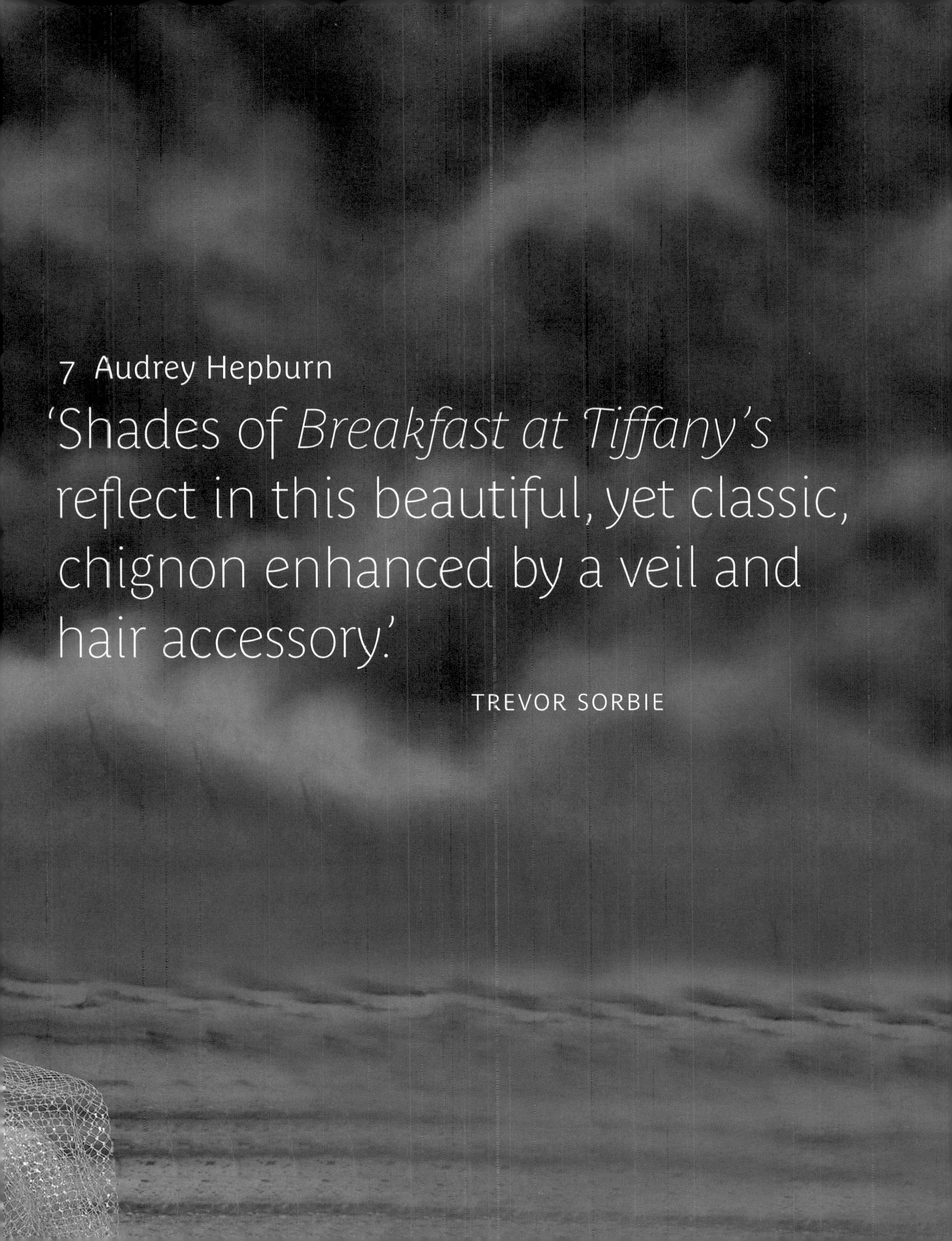

7 Audrey Hepburn

'Shades of *Breakfast at Tiffany's* reflect in this beautiful, yet classic, chignon enhanced by a veil and hair accessory.'

TREVOR SORBIE

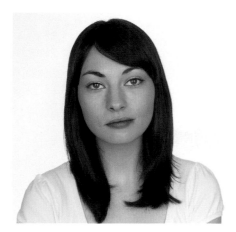

1 Before.

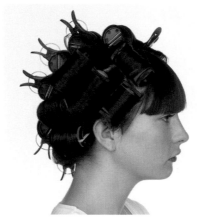

2 Set hair on heated rollers, leaving out the fringe.

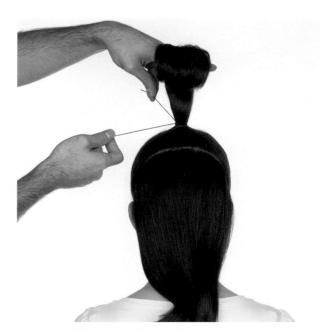

3 Remove rollers, section hair as shown and tie crown hair into a ponytail.

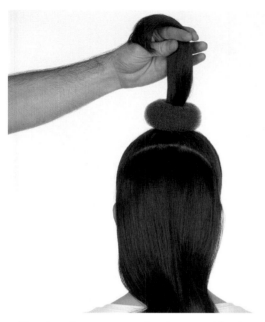

4 Place bun ring over ponytail and secure with grips.

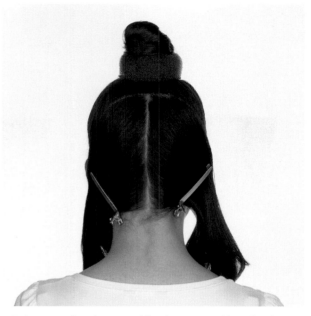

5 Twist ponytail and secure with grips on top of bun ring for the time being. Part hair down centre back.

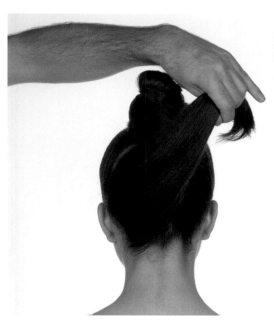

6 Smooth one back section with a bristle brush, wrapping ends around bun ring. Grip in place. Repeat with other back section, smoothing around the bun ring.

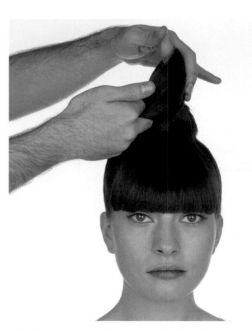

7 Release reserved hair from topknot and shape over bun, then secure with grips.

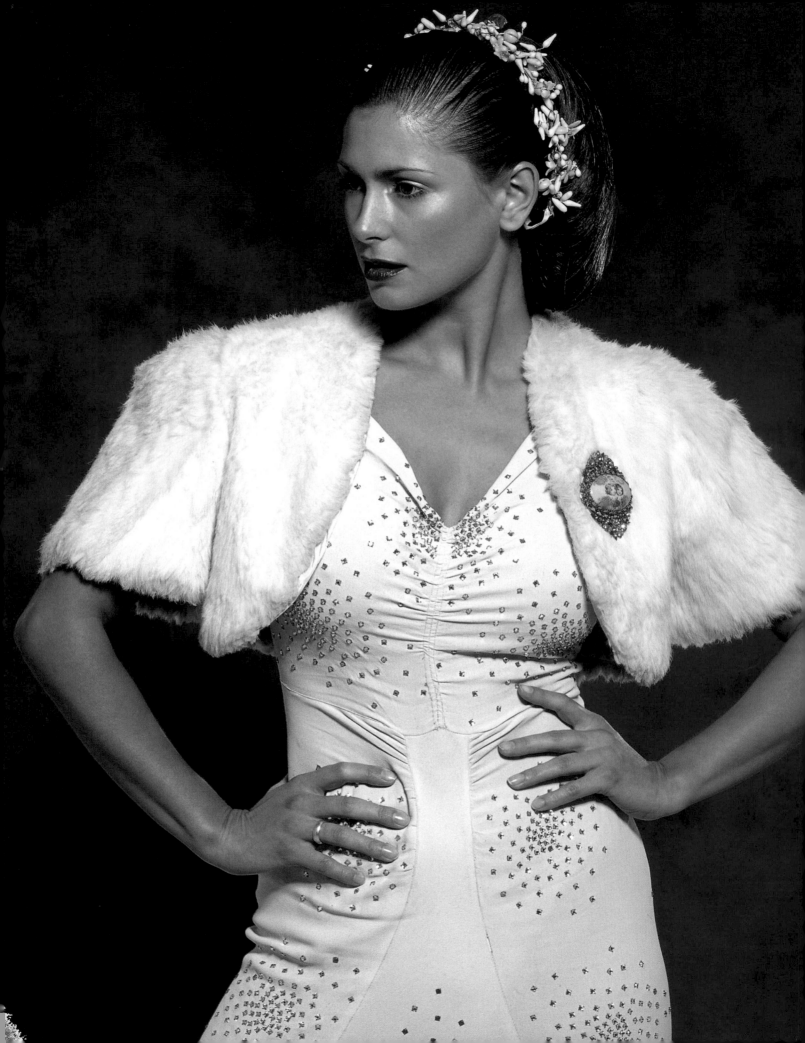

'For the traditionalist, a simple swept-back look which is then backcombed to give a voluminous shape.'

TREVOR SORBIE

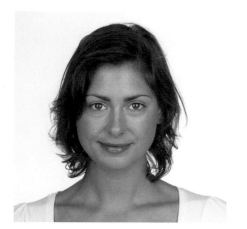

1 Before.

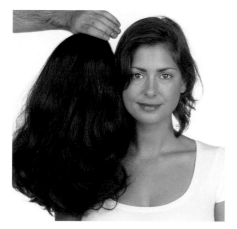

2 Match hairpiece to colour of hair.

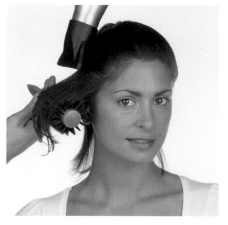

3 Blow dry hair smooth using a round bristle brush.

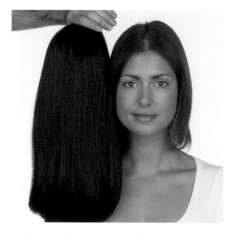

4 Blow dry hairpiece smooth.

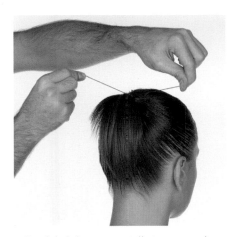

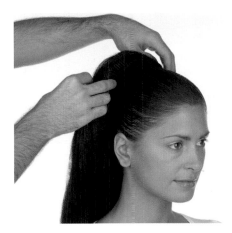

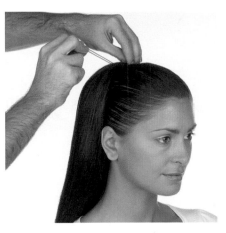

5 Brush hair into a ponytail at crown and secure with elastic.

6 Secure comb of hairpiece on top of ponytail.

7 Secure with pins.

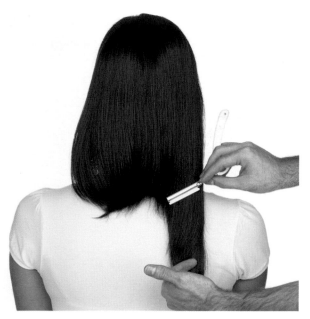

8 Remove excess length from hairpiece using a razor.

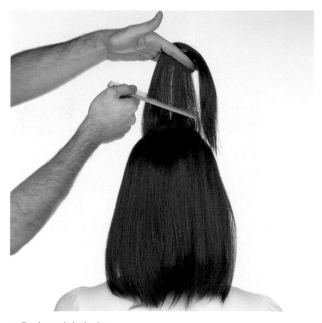

9 Backcomb hairpiece.

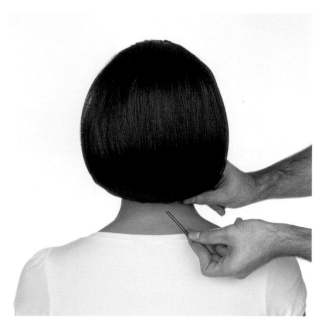

10 Smooth over using a bristle brush, tuck in ends and pin at nape.

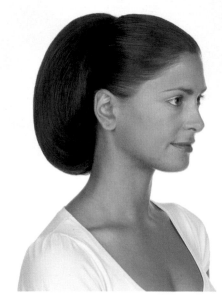

11 Shows side view.

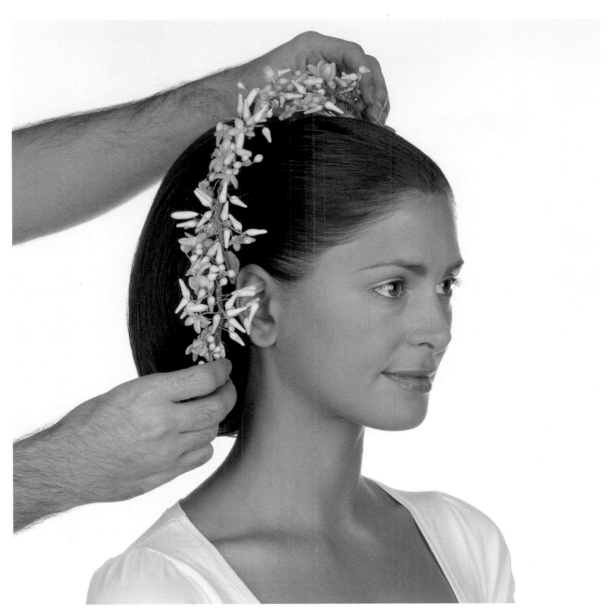

12 Add hair accessory and secure in place with grips.

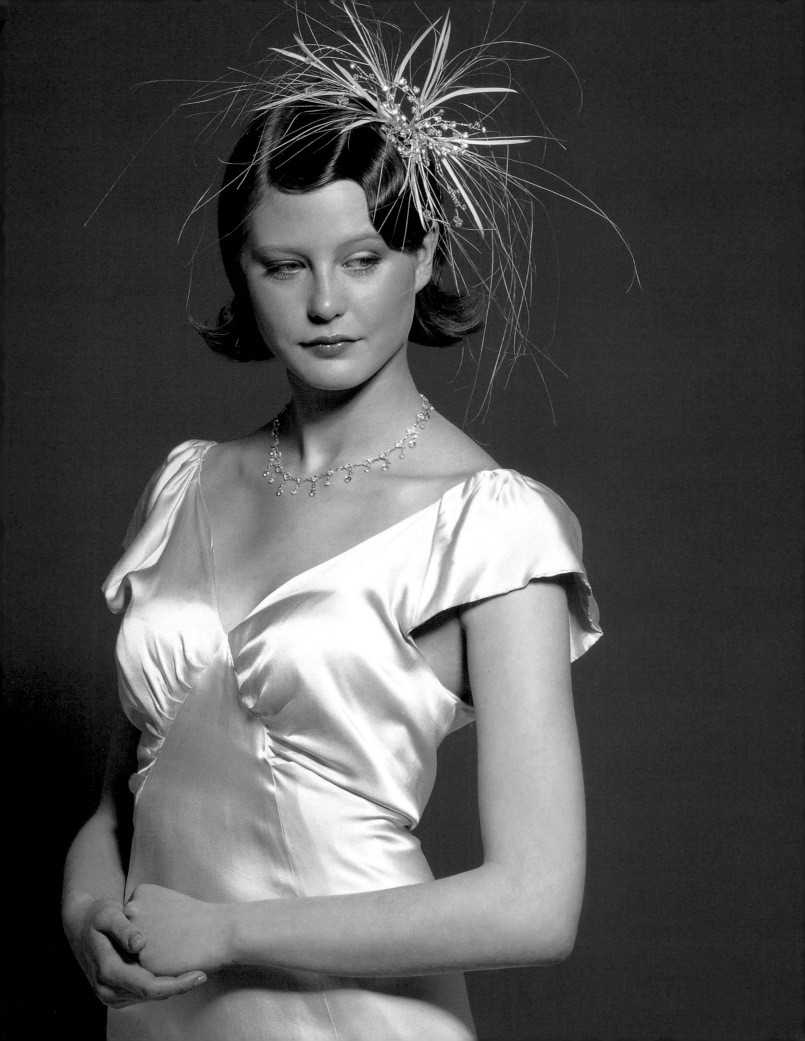

9 Finger Waves

'Using a traditional finger-waving
technique in the front coupled
with flick-ups at the back, we get
a fresh approach to a classic look.'

TREVOR SORBIE

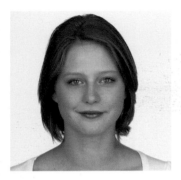

1 Before.

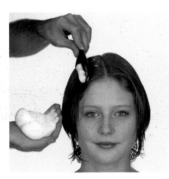

2 Apply mousse using a wide toothcomb.

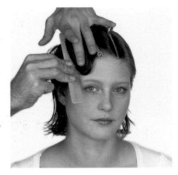

3 Part hair at side and use comb to finger-wave front hair, pushing wave into place with fingers and comb to form an S shape.

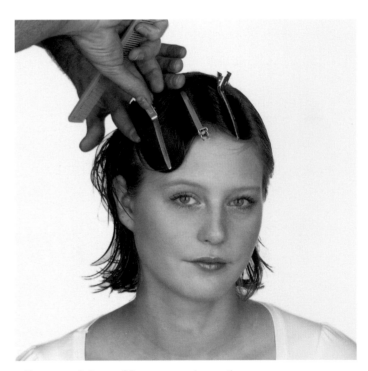

4 Form next S shape of finger-wave using section clips in crest of waves to keep in place.

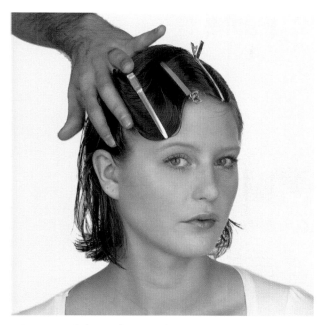

5 Form next S shape of wave and insert section clip.

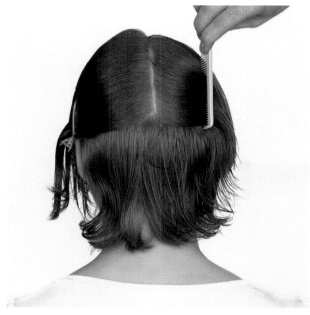

6 Part hair as shown.

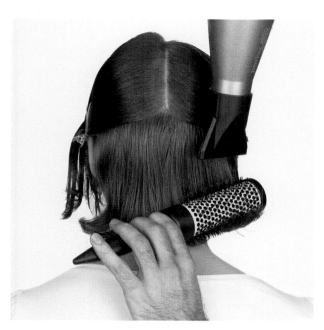

7 Blow dry lower hair using a ceramic round bristle brush, flicking out er ds. Blow dry top hair.

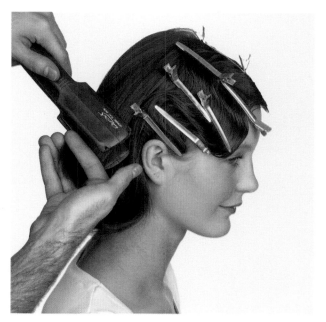

8 Straighten top layers of hair further using smoothing irons, then diffuser dry finger-waves before removing clips.

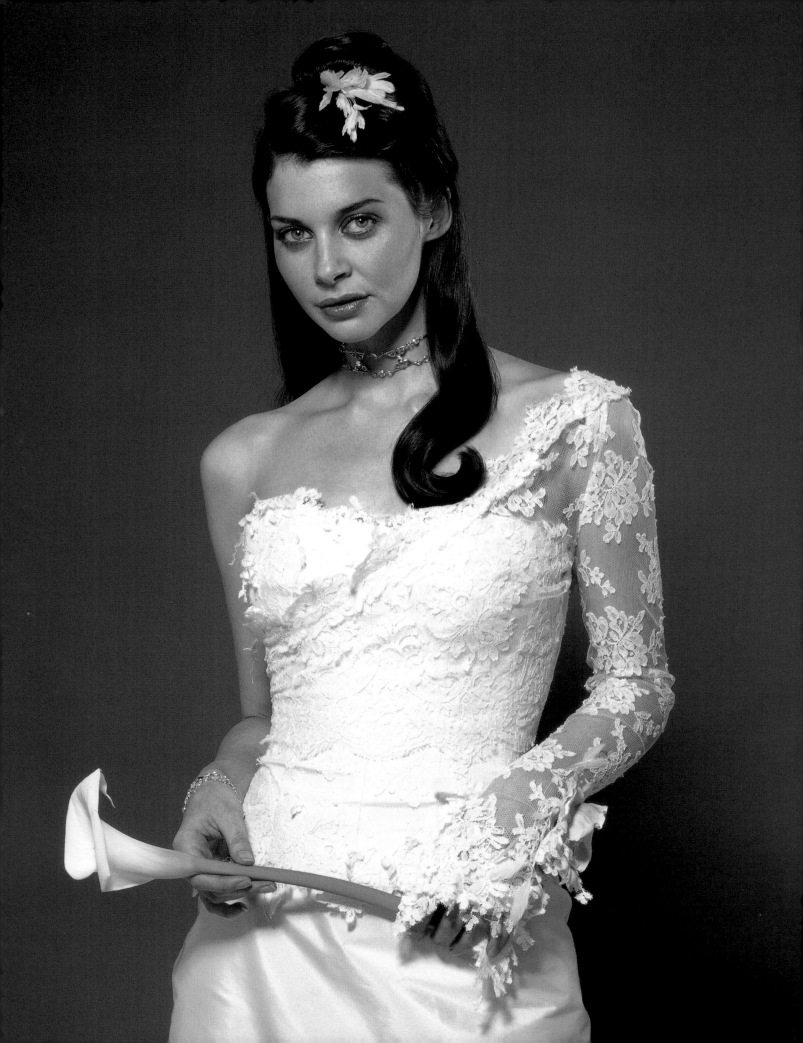

'For brides who still want to have the feeling of long hair this simple half up, half down classic look is a winner.'

TREVOR SORBIE

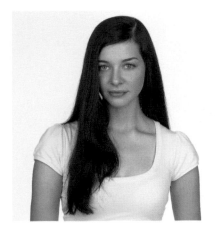

1 Before.

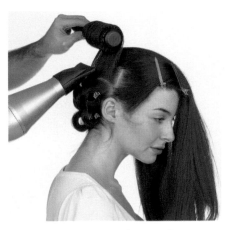

2 Damp hair with pre-style spray then blow dry using a ceramic round brush.

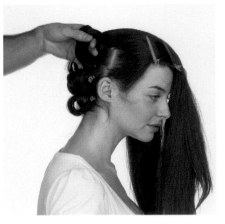

3 As you finish drying each section, roll into a barrel curl.

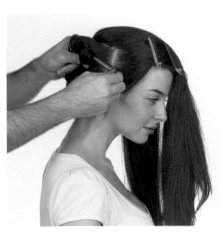

4 Use a section clip to hold in place.

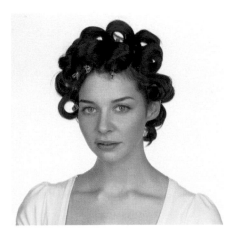

5 Shows completed barrel curl pli.

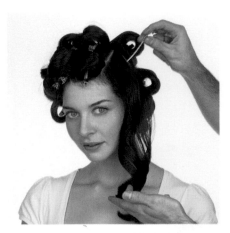

6 Remove section clips and let hair fall free.

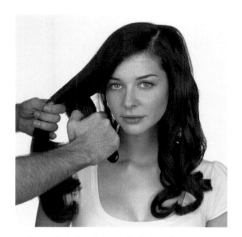

7 Smooth hair with a bristle brush.

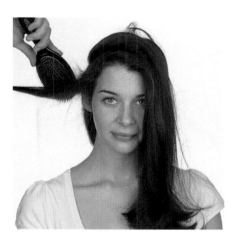

8 Back brush from ear on one side to side parting on other side.

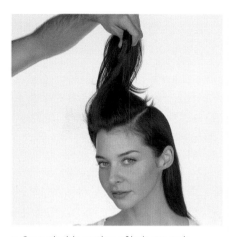

9 Smooth this section of hair upwards and twist clockwise.

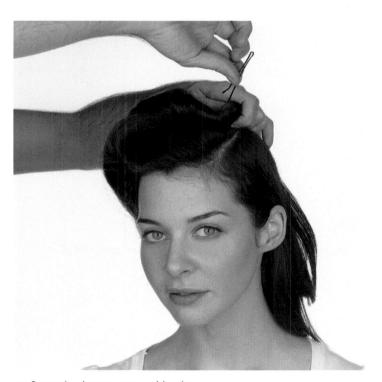

10 Secure in place on crown with grips. Brush lower hair onto shoulders to form a soft wave.

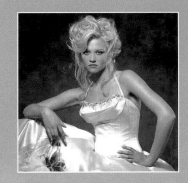
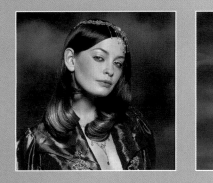
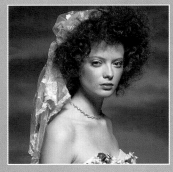
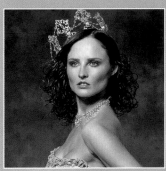

GLAMOROUS

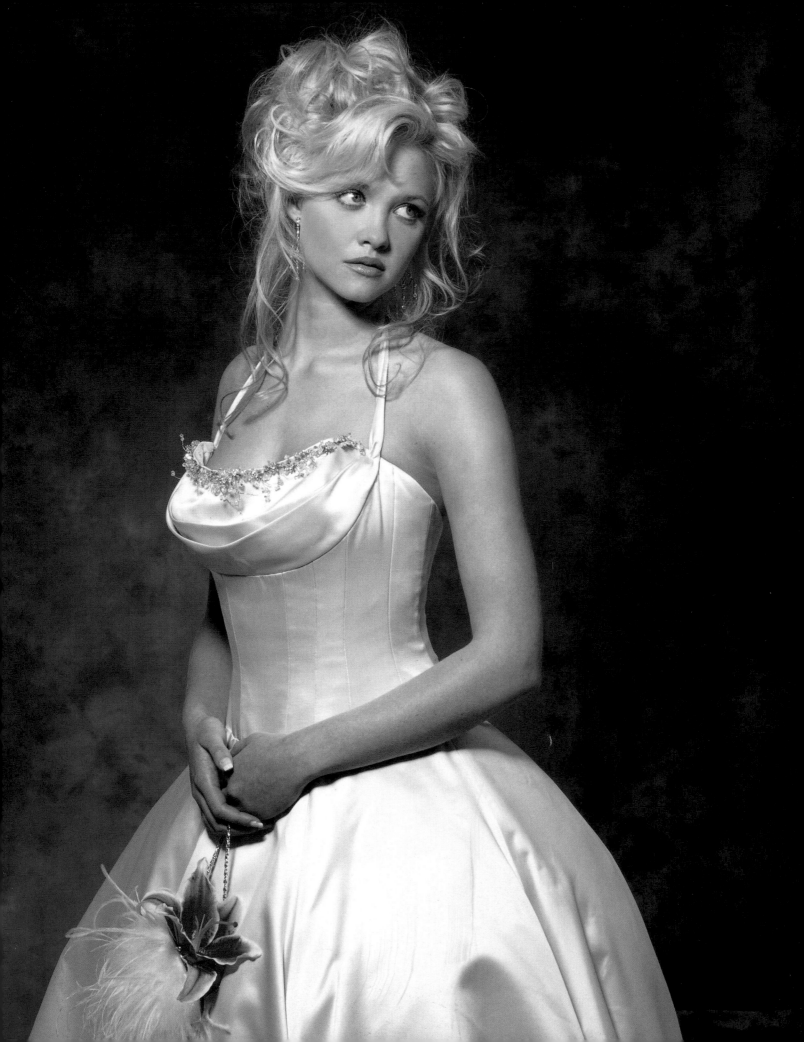

11 Bridget Bardot

'The model's face reminded me
of Bridget Bardot so we gave her
a tousled, dishevelled look that is
"oh so sexy".'

TREVOR SORBIE

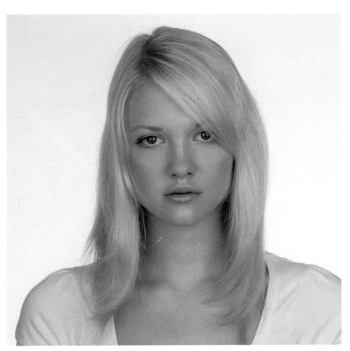

1 Before.

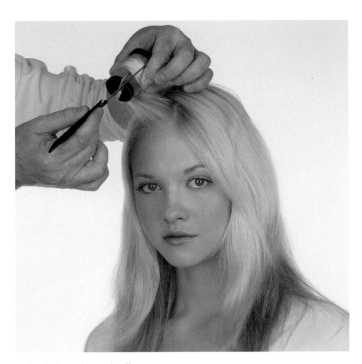

2 Set hair on heated rollers.

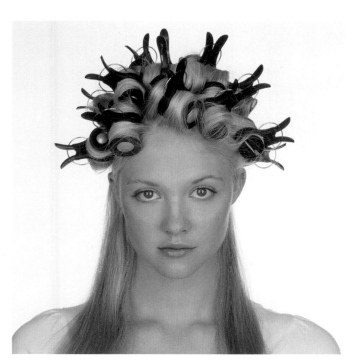

3 Shows top hair set on heated rollers. Continue setting lower ha r.

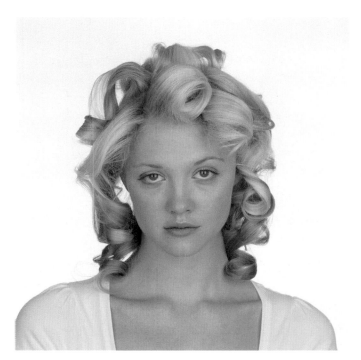

4 When hair is cold remove heated rollers.

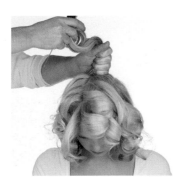

5 Take a 7.5cm section at crown.

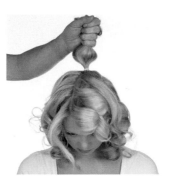

6 Secure into a ponytail with a band.

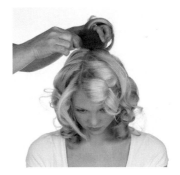

7 Insert bun ring over ponytail, and grip in place.

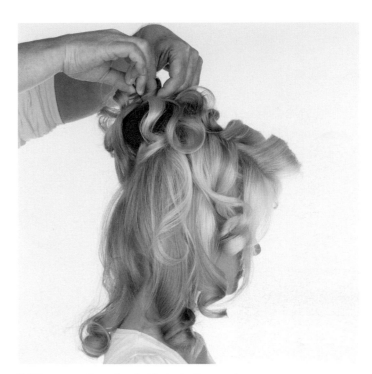

8 Take one section of curled hair at a time and grip in to place at random on the bun ring. Leave some tendrils to fall free.

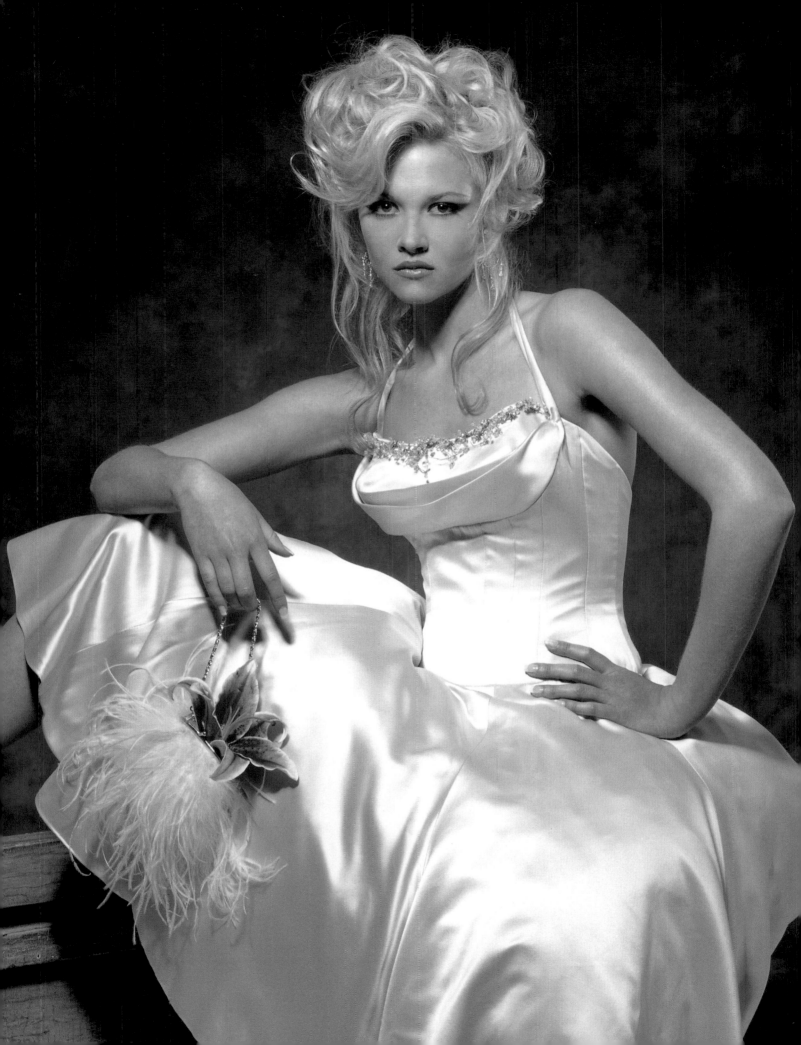

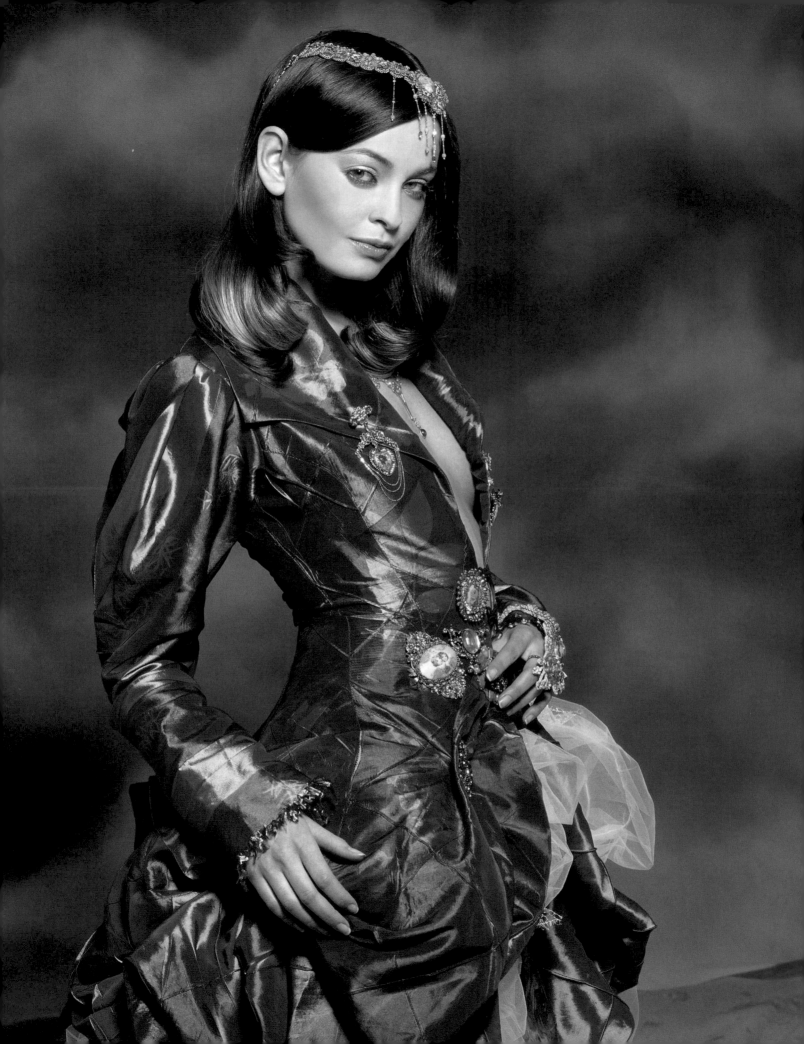

12 Coloured Wefts

'The hair itself is simple but what makes it amazing is the clever use of a coloured weft incorporated into the hair which is echoed by the stunning gown.'

TREVOR SORBIE

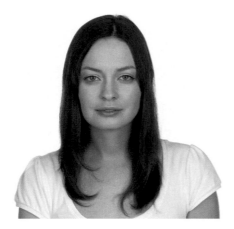

1 Before.

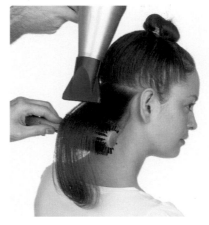

2 Section hair then blow dry lower hair using a round bristle brush.

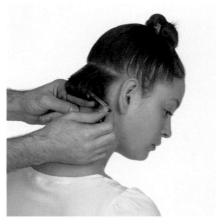

3 Form hair into a large barrel curl and use section clip to secure at nape.

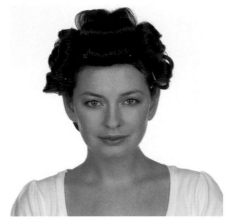

4 Shows completed blow dry with each section clipped into a barrel curl.

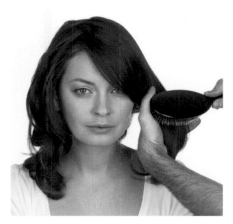

5 Remove clips and smooth hair with a bristle brush.

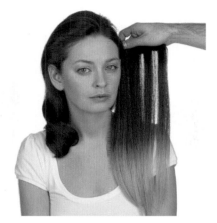

6 Hold weft up to check length.

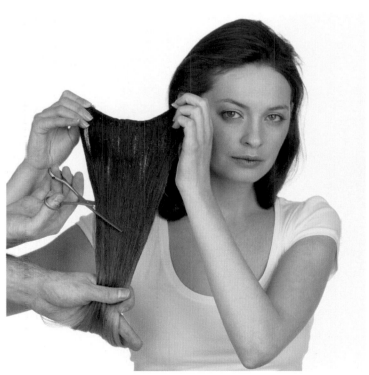

7 Use thinning scissors to remove weight and length from weft.

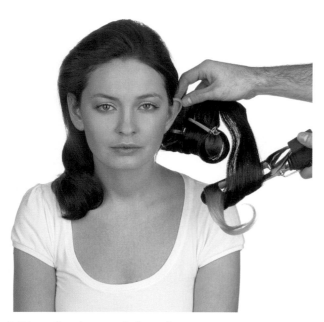

8 Take weft and tong and clip to give movement.

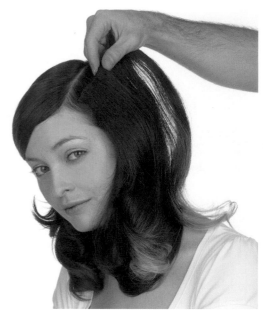

9 Part hair at side and position weft parallel to parting.

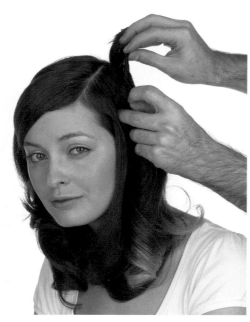

10 Use specialist clips attached to top of weft to secure weft in place along parting.

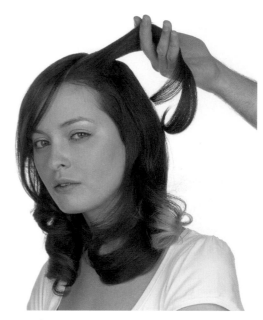

11 Take a section from crown parallel to parting and comb over weft to hide base. Smooth hair and weft together with a bristle bush.

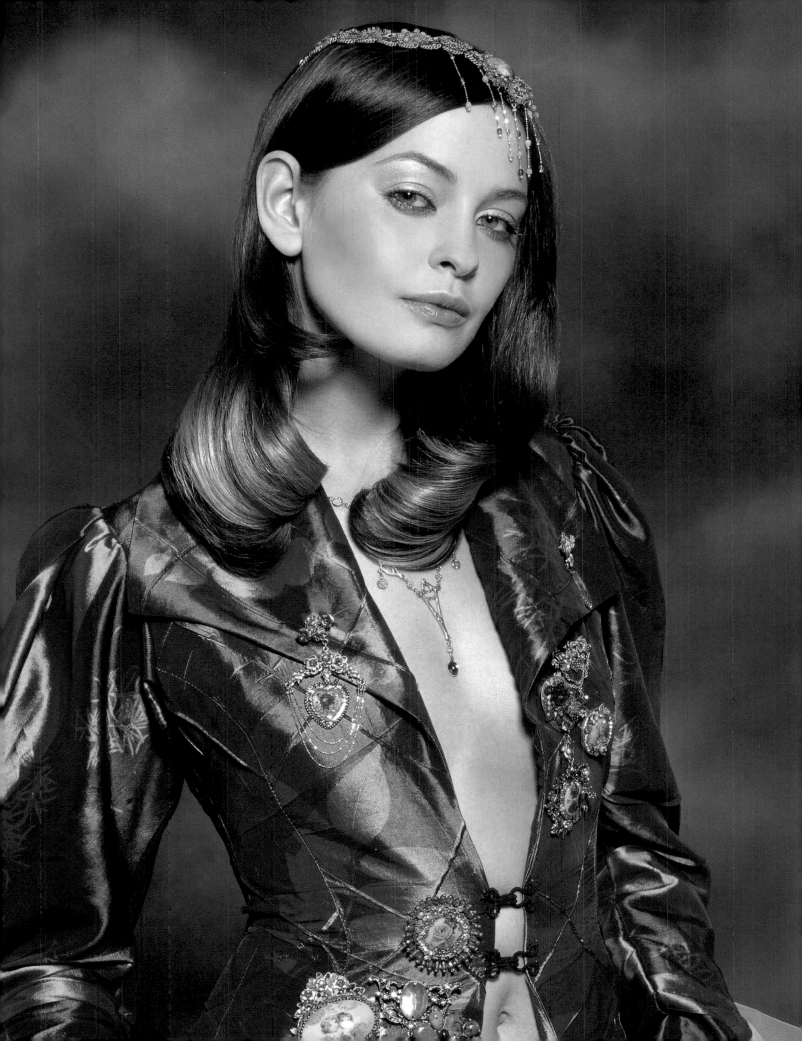

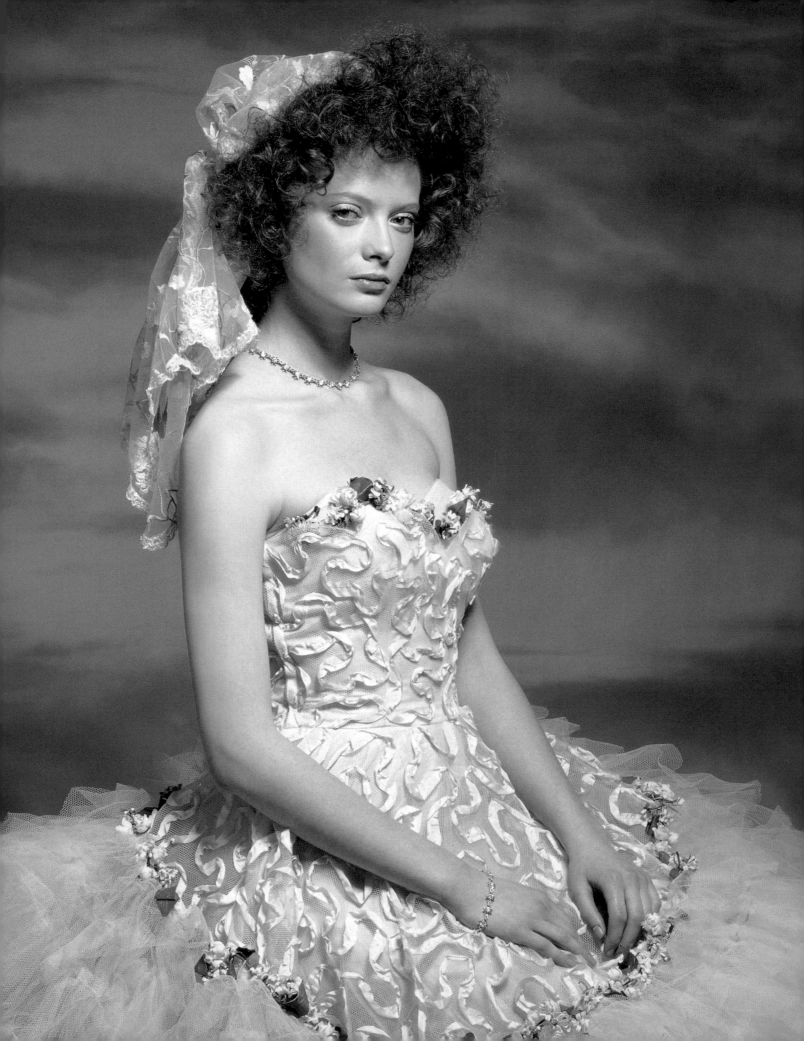

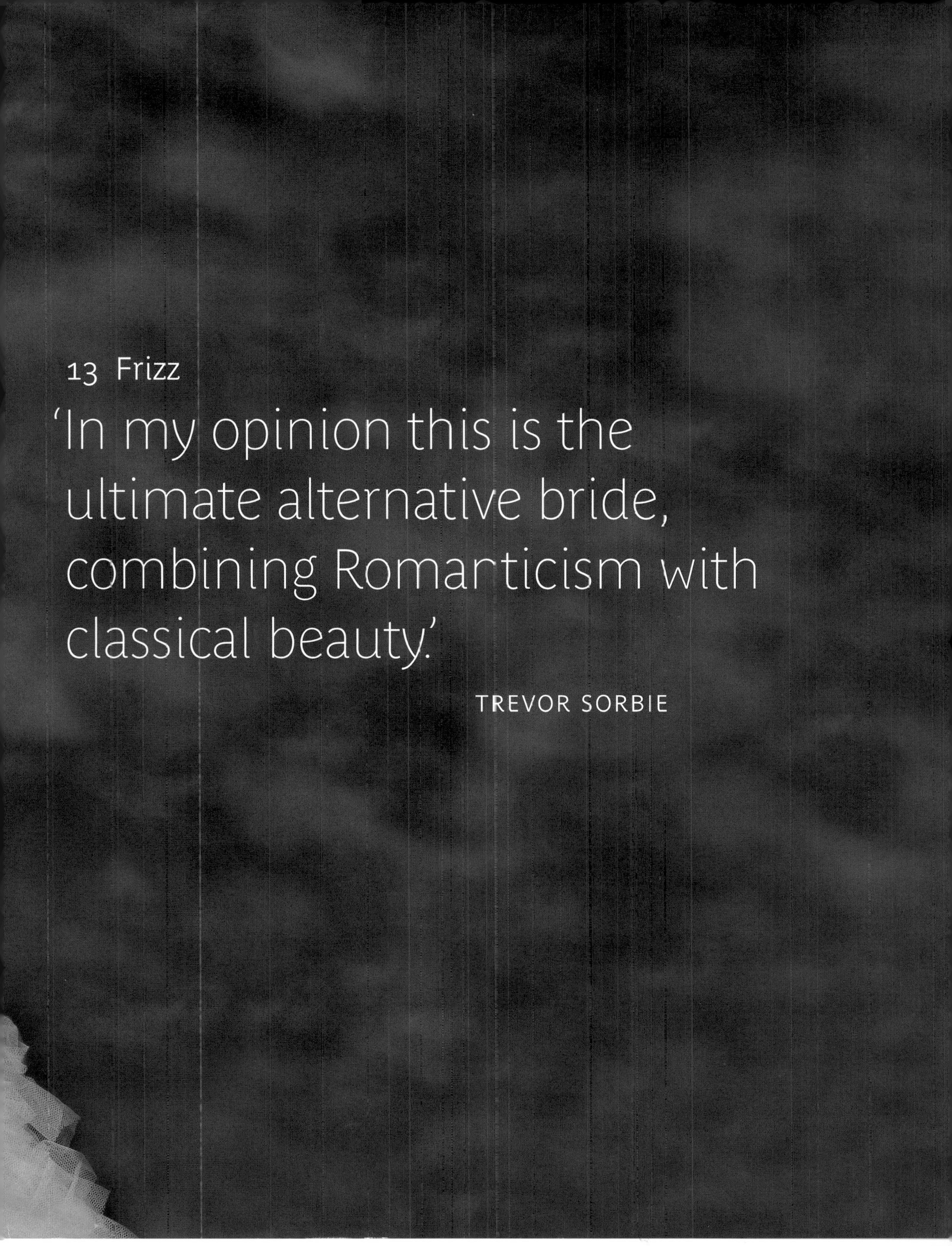

13 Frizz

'In my opinion this is the ultimate alternative bride, combining Romarticism with classical beauty.'

TREVOR SORBIE

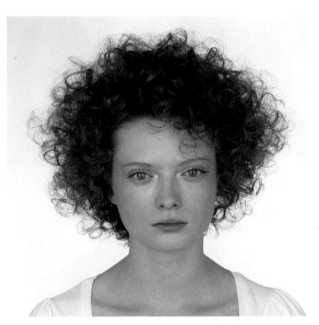

7 Shows hair back brushed with thumb and forefinger.

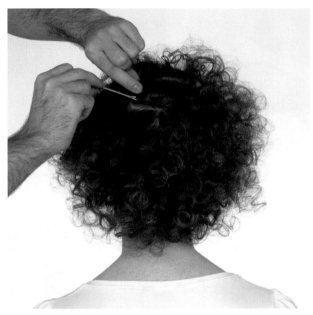

8 At back, fold over and pin a section of hair to form a 'pad' to attach veil with grips. This means it will be more secure and will not loosen or fall out.

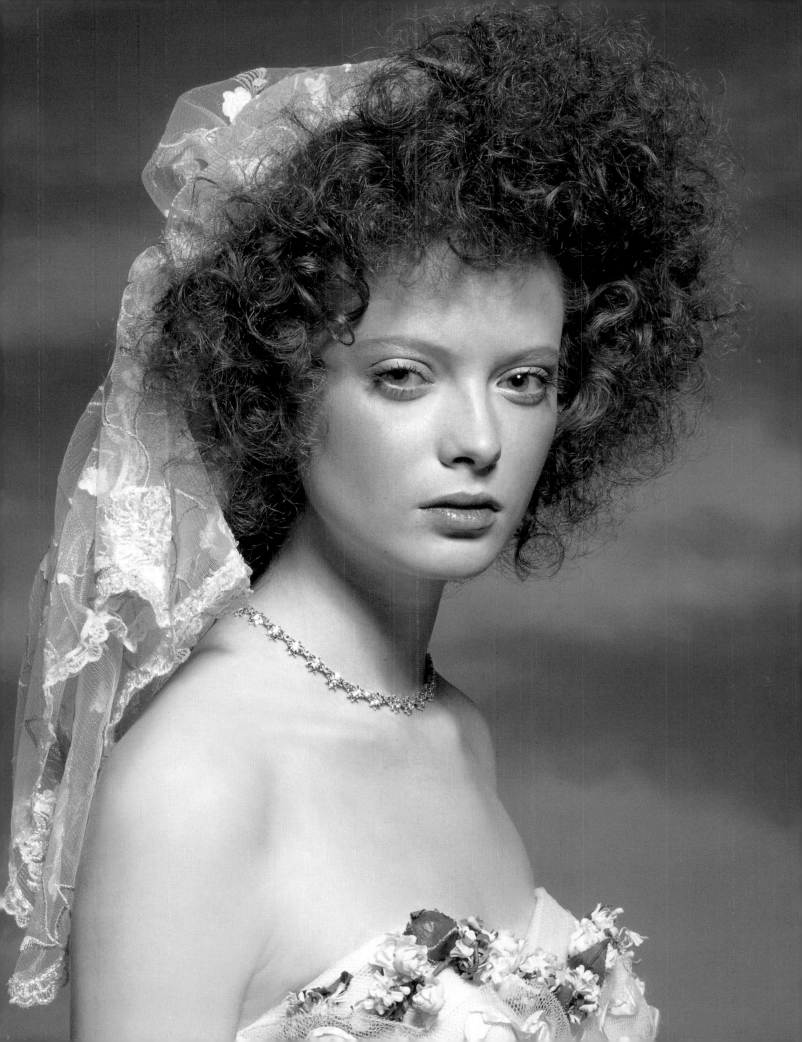

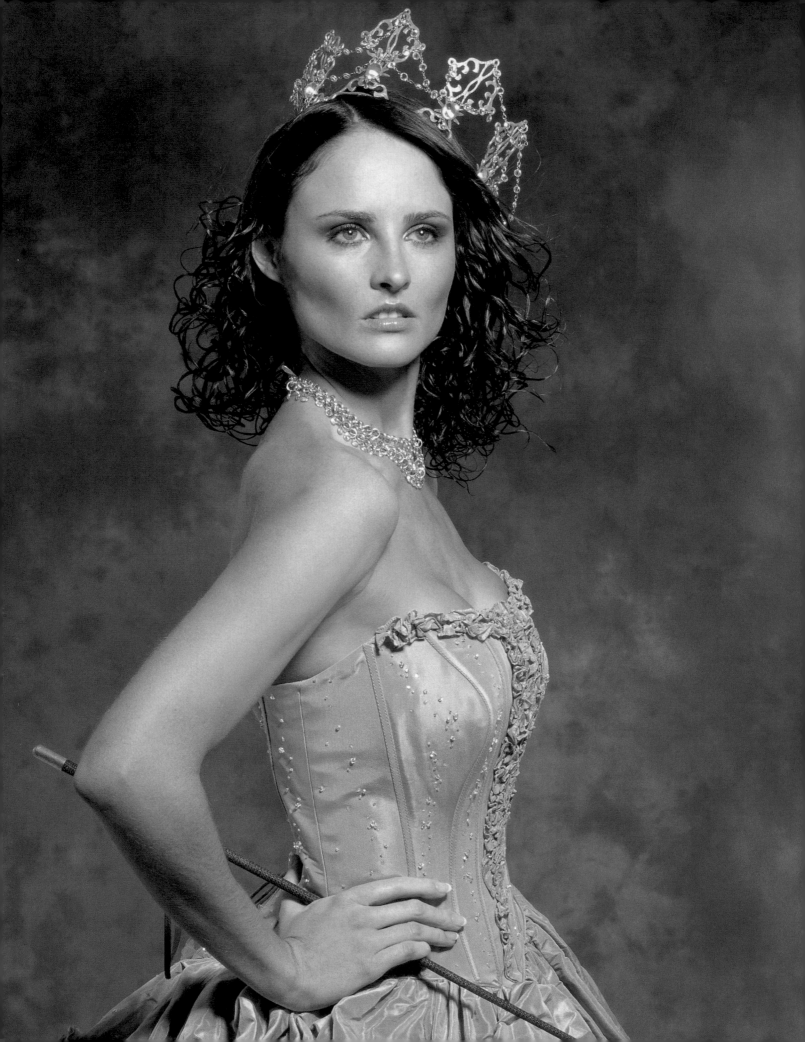

'Twisting small sections of hair and diffuser drying gives this lovely twig-like texture to naturally wavy hair.'

TREVOR SORBIE

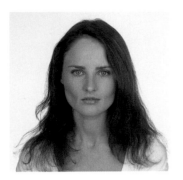

1 Before.

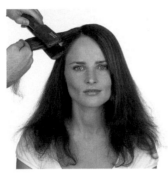

2 Straighten hair from top to eye level at sides and crown to occipital bone at back using smoothing irons. Leave lower hair unstraightened.

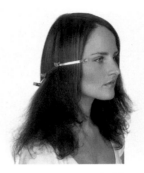

3 Use section clips to hold straightened hair in place.

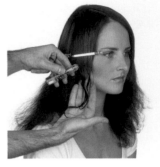

4 Soak a small section of hair with setting lotion.

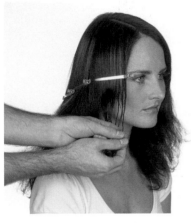

5 Divide into fine strands and twist each one.

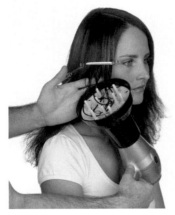

6 Gently diffuser dry using low heat and speed setting. Allow hair to dry undisturbed in the diffuser cup.

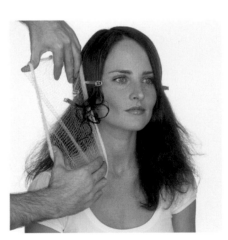

7 Place these dried curls in a hairnet to hold, then work on remaining lower hair in same way. Place each section in a net after drying. This protects the curls from being disturbed by the airflow as you work round.

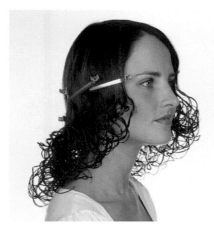

8 Shows all lower hair curled with hair net removed.

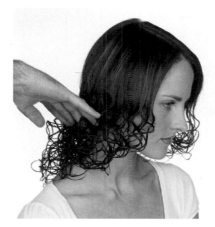

9 Gently loosen hair using fingers.

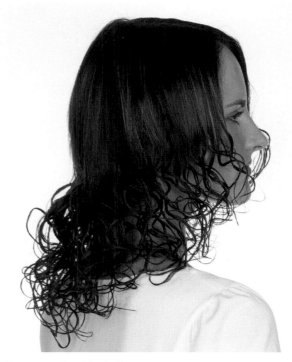

10 Shows completed back view.

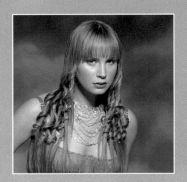

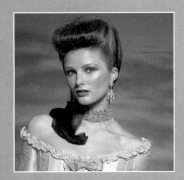

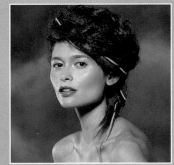

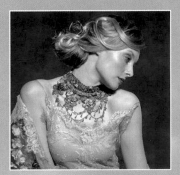

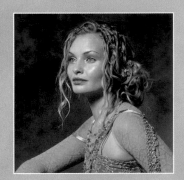

ROMANTIC

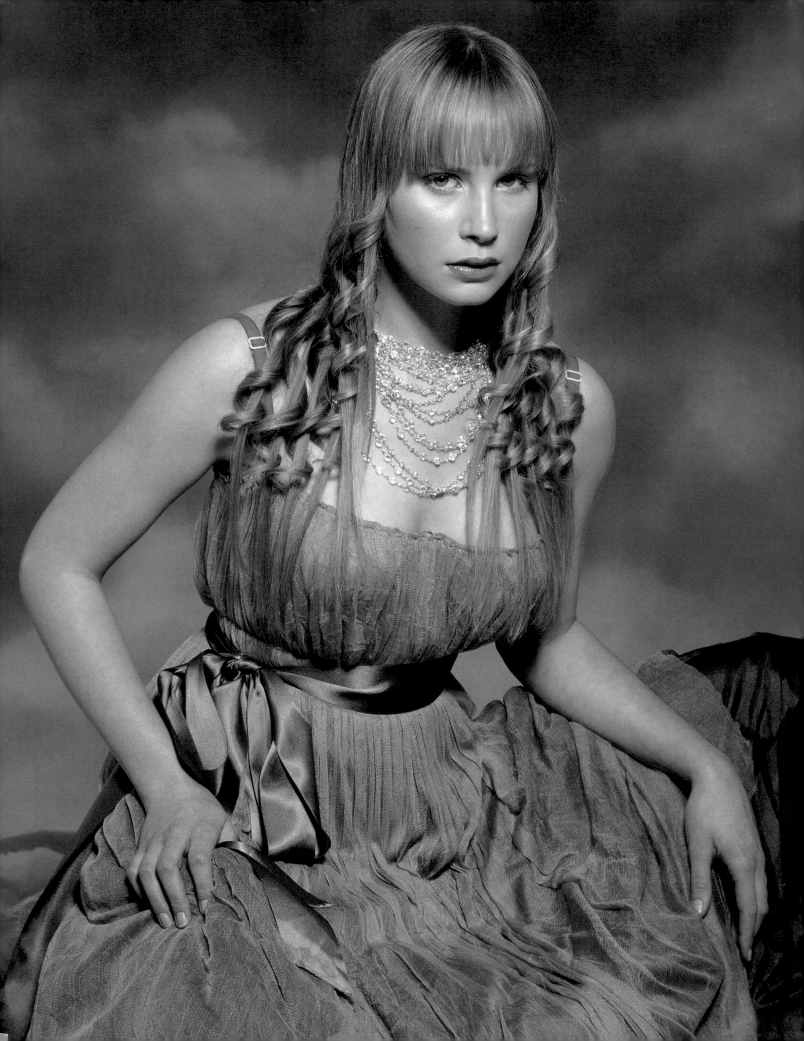

15 Spiral Curls

'Using a simple technique of curling hair around straight hair gives an unusual but beautiful twist on wearing long hair down.'

TREVOR SORBIE

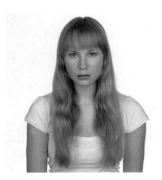

1 Before.

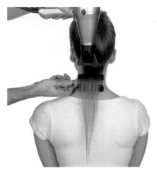

2 Blow dry hair smooth starting at nape and using a round bristle brush. Do not overheat the hair or tonging will not take.

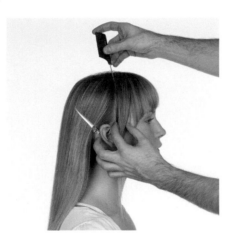

3 Take first section at front, then clip remaining hair back using a section clip.

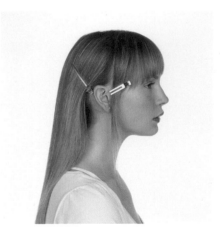

4 Shows first section.

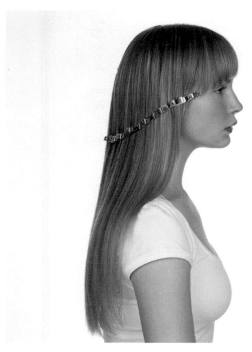

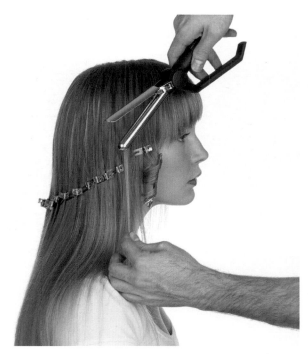

5 Continue making sections, clipping each as you work, right round head. This guideline should graduate from eye level down to nape as shown.

6 Hold tong horizontally and tong first section, holding the curl using a section clip. Leave one section straight. Then tong next section.

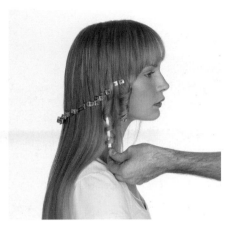

7 Clip section as before and continue in same way.

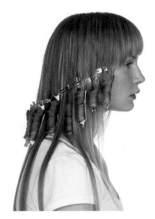

8 Continue working in same way all round head, i.e. tonging, clipping a section, missing a section and repeating.

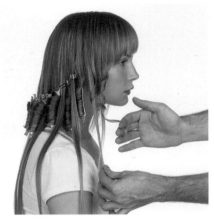

9 Take first tonged section and wrap round straight section. Repeat all round head.

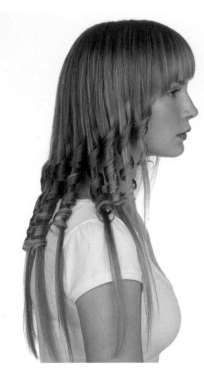

10 Shows completed tonged curls twirled round straight sections.

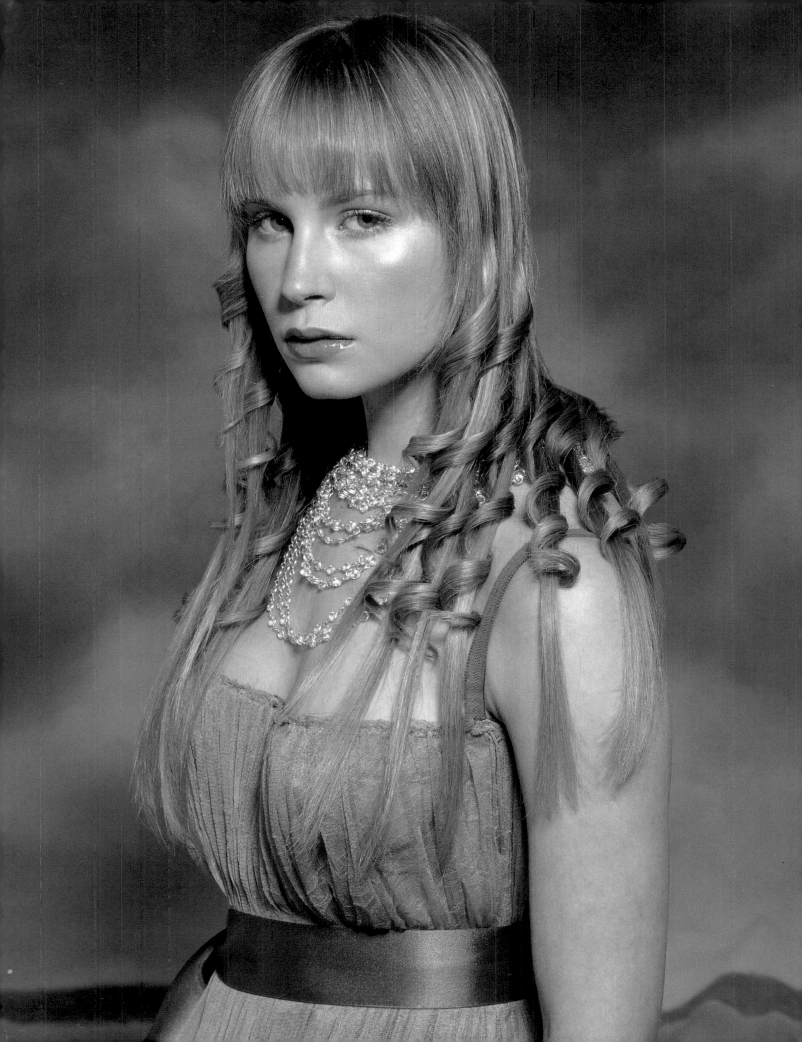

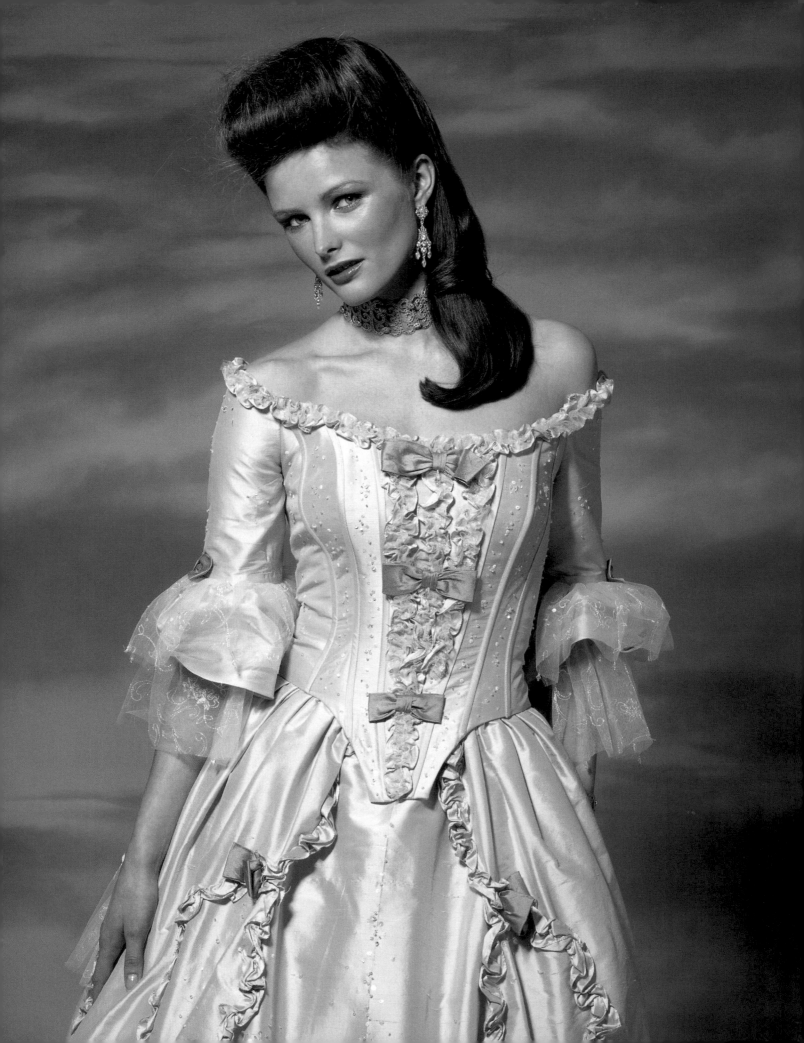

16 Scarlett O'Hara

'Inspired by Scarlett O'Hara, this look encapsulates the essence of a bygone era when hair accentuated the beautiful shape of the gowns.'

TREVOR SORBIE

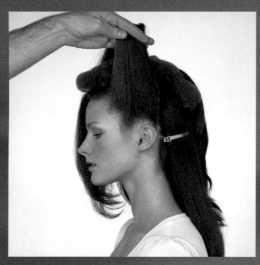

9 Take side section of hair and brush upwards to centre of crown. Secure with pin in bun ring.

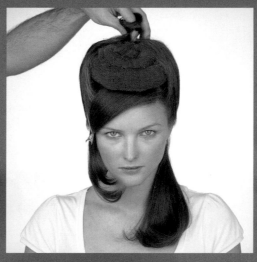

10 Repeat with other side section of hair, and pin in place.

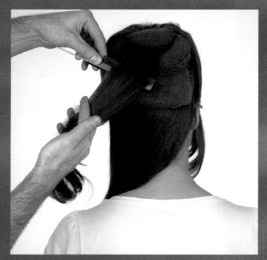

11 Take reserved hair from centre ponytail, backcomb and smooth over and around bun ring, and pin in place.

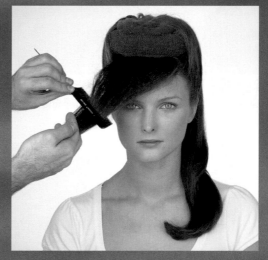

12 Take front reserved hair, backcomb, smooth upwards to cover remaining uncovered parts of bun ring.

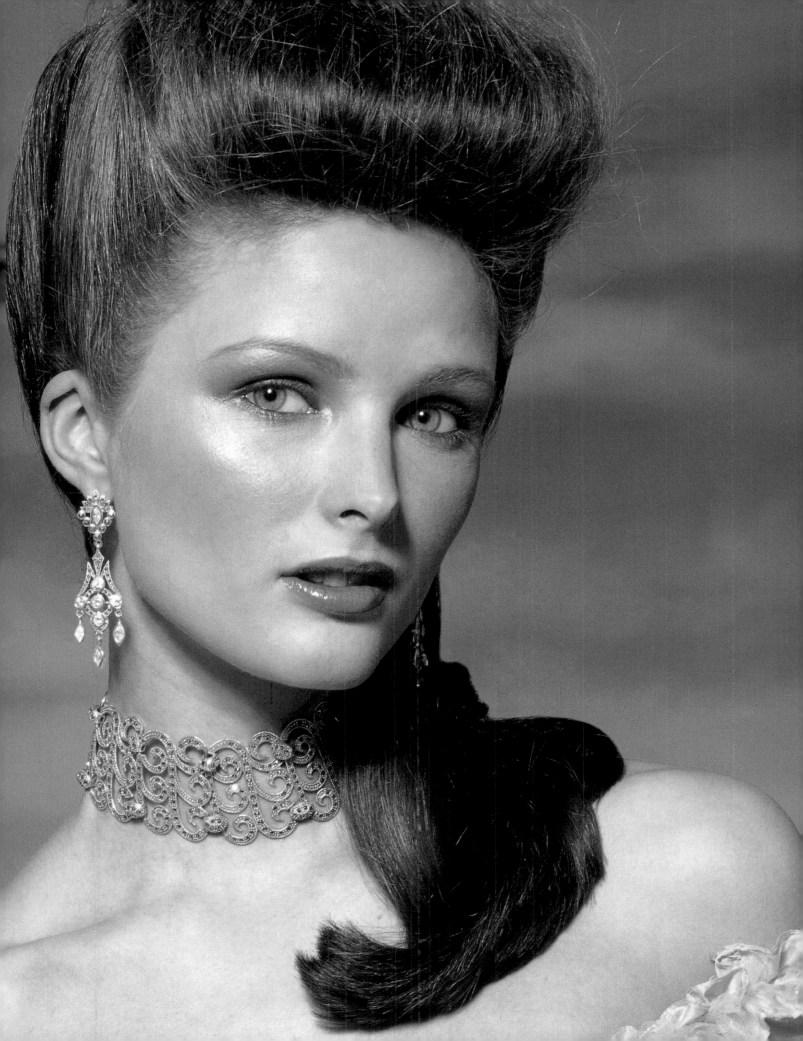

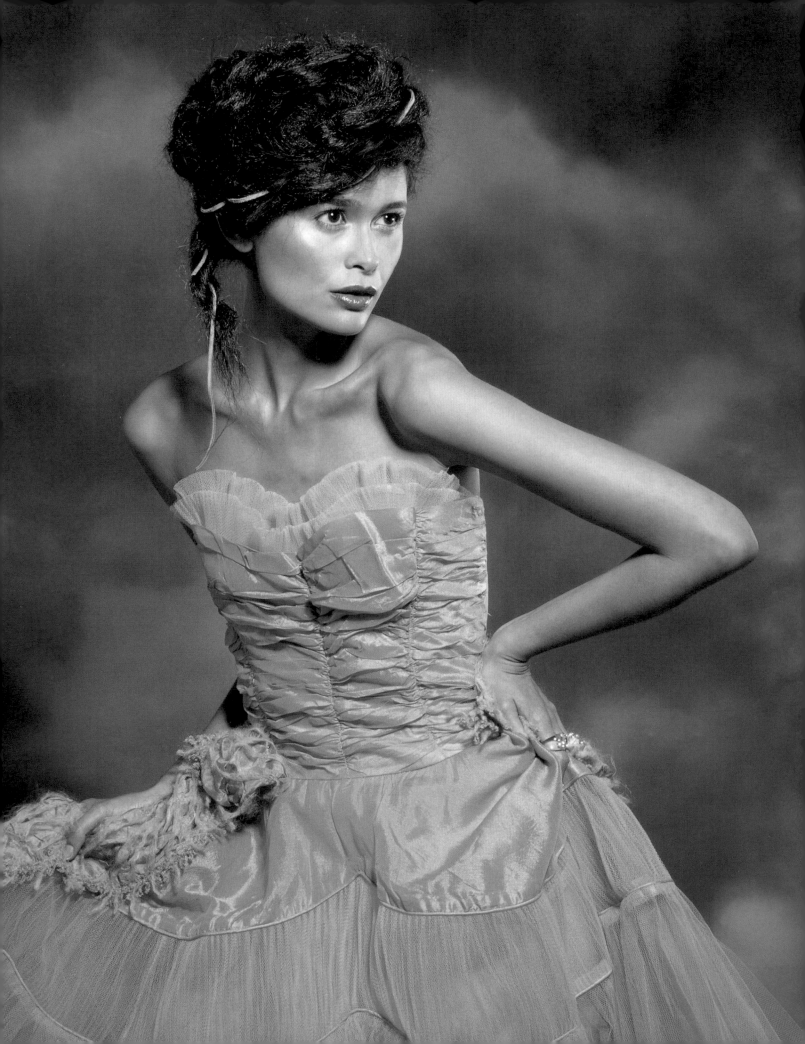

17 Dreadlocks

'Dreadlocks are used in an unusual way to show how street fashion can be interpreted for that ultimate occasion.'

TREVOR SORBIE

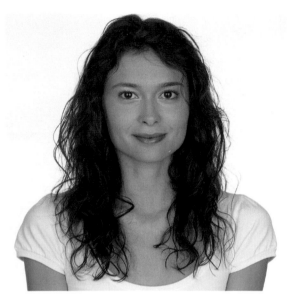

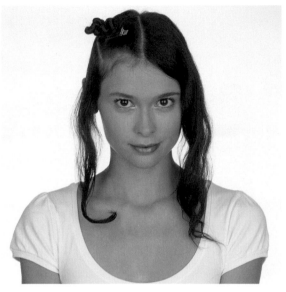

1 Before.

2 Part hair in centre. Clip back hair out of the way. Take a 5 cm square section from one side of parting. Twist hair until it doubles back on itself and clip.

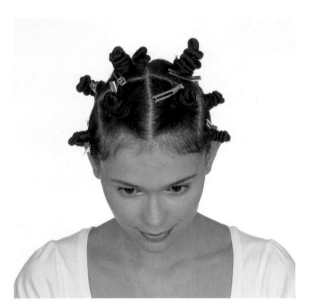

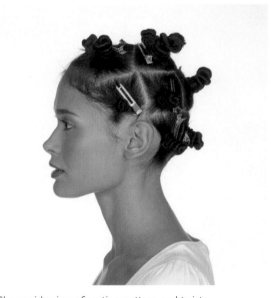

3 Twist remaining hair in same way. This shows the front view.

4 Shows side view of section pattern and twists.

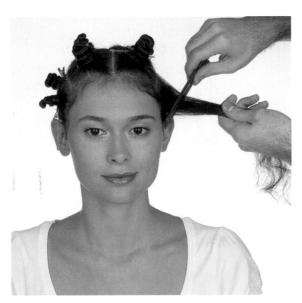

5 Take one section and backcomb from roots to ends.

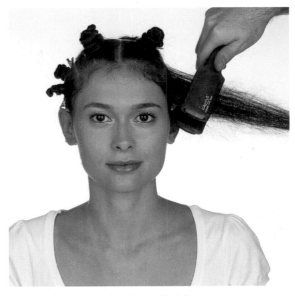

6 Clamp backcombed section of hair between smoothing irons.

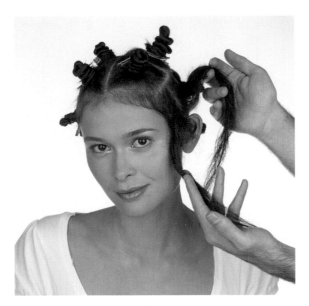

7 Split backcombed section into two.

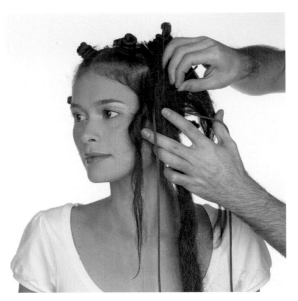

8 Place leather and dreadlock in place between back-combed section and secure with grip. You should have an equal length of dreadlock and leather on either side.

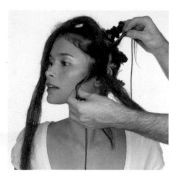

9 Cross leather and natural hair over dreadlock.

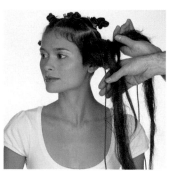

10 Divide so you have second section of leather/dreadlock and natural hair, then twist together to form a rope.

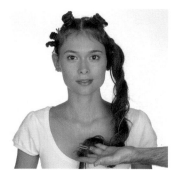

11 Secure at bottom of dreadlock with a clip.

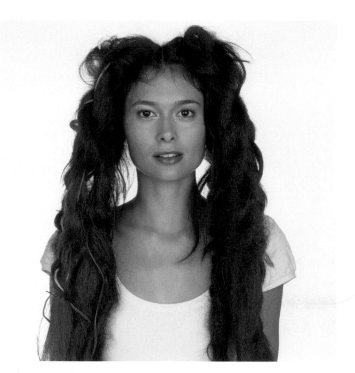

12 Shows dreadlocks in place. Now twist and pile up and pin to top of head.

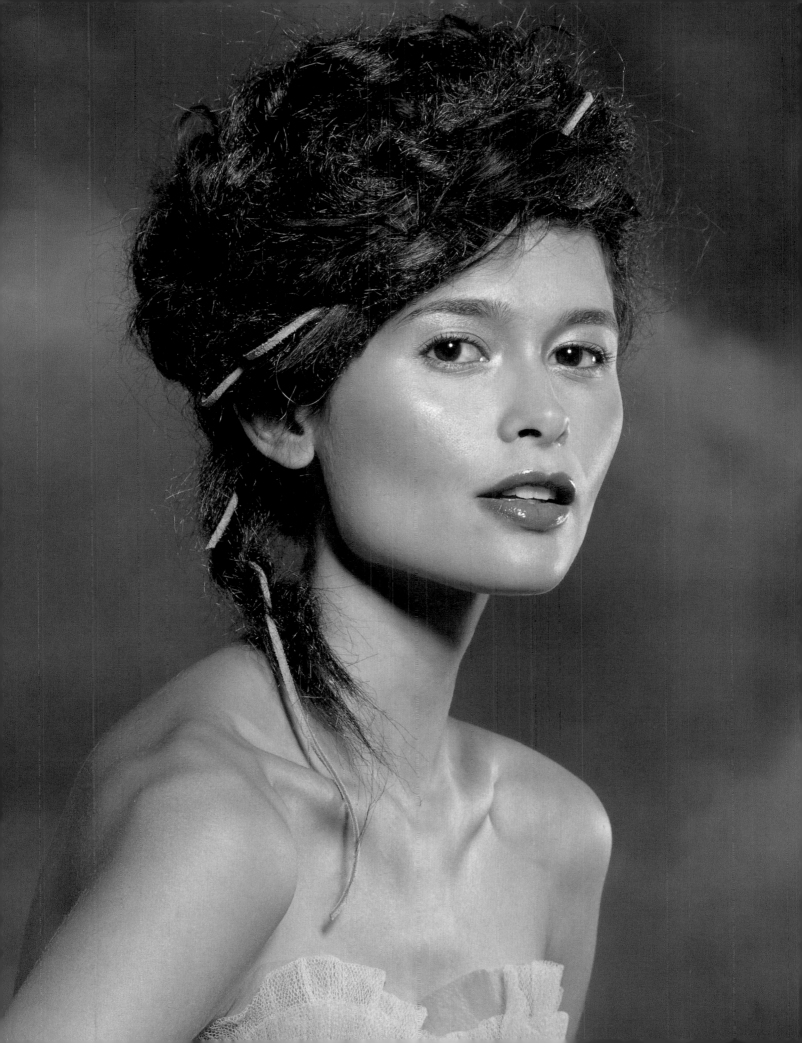

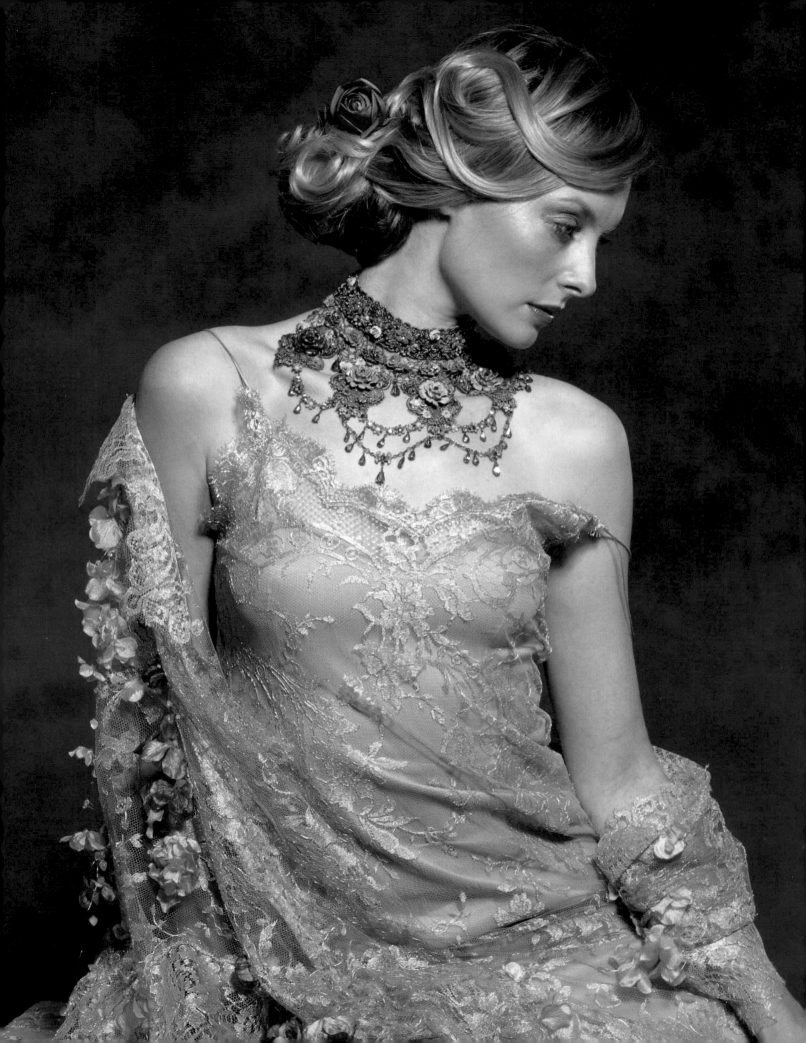

18 Coils

'The inspiration for this look was taken from the Pre-Raphaelite era and has been complemented by this stunning gown and necklace.'

TREVOR SORBIE

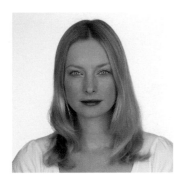

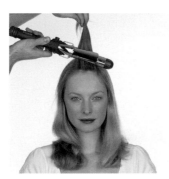

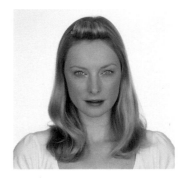

1 Before.

2 Smooth first section of hair with large tongs.

3 Set in a barrel curl. Continue working in this way.

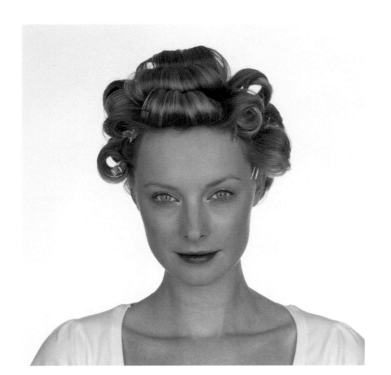

4 Shows completed barrel curl pli.

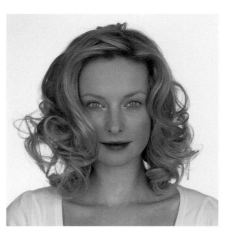

5 Remove clips and let curls fall.

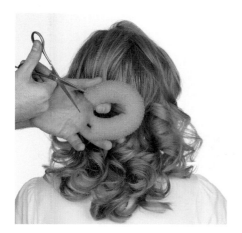

6 Take a bun ring and cut as shown. Repeat with another bun ring.

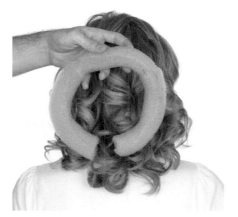

7 Pin the two pieces of cut bun ring together as shown.

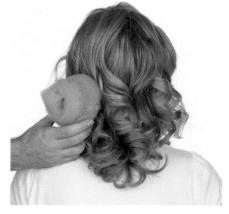

8 Form bun ring into a cone and pin to hold shape. Picture shows where bun ring will be positioned later.

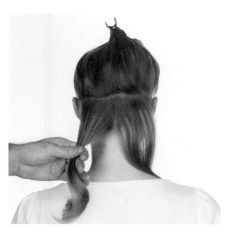

9 Section hair as shown.

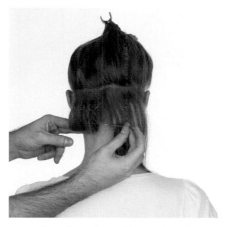

10 Backcomb section, roll into a barrel curl and pin.

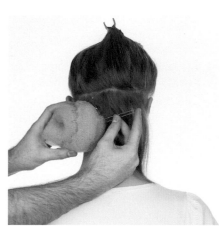

11 Pin bun ring in position.

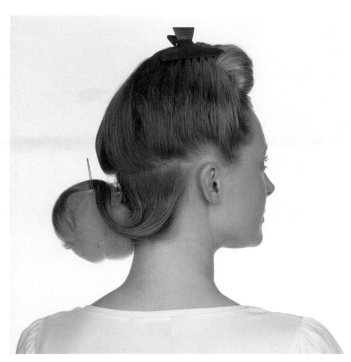

12 Take other nape section of hair, form into a wave and position on top of bun ring.

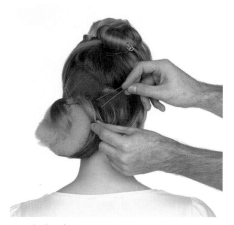

13 Pin in place.

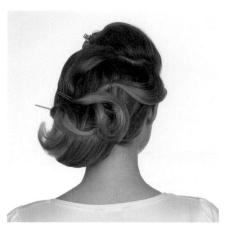

14 Continue working this way, taking sections from clipped up hair, forming wavy swirls and pinning in place.

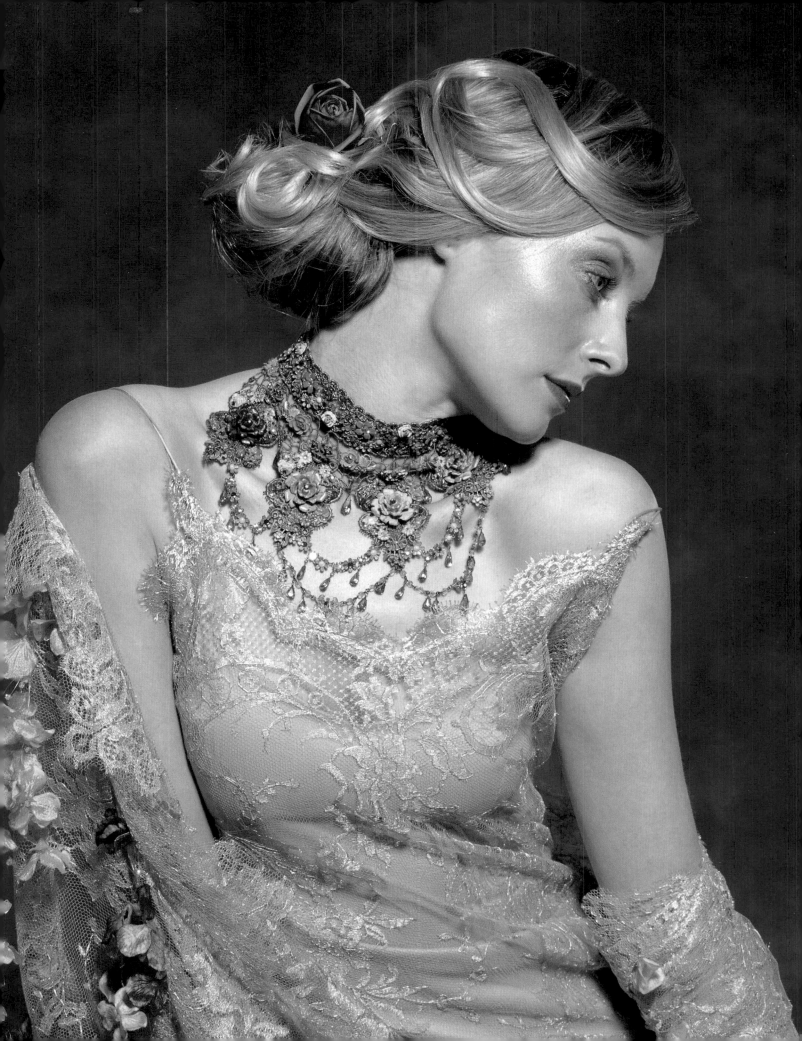

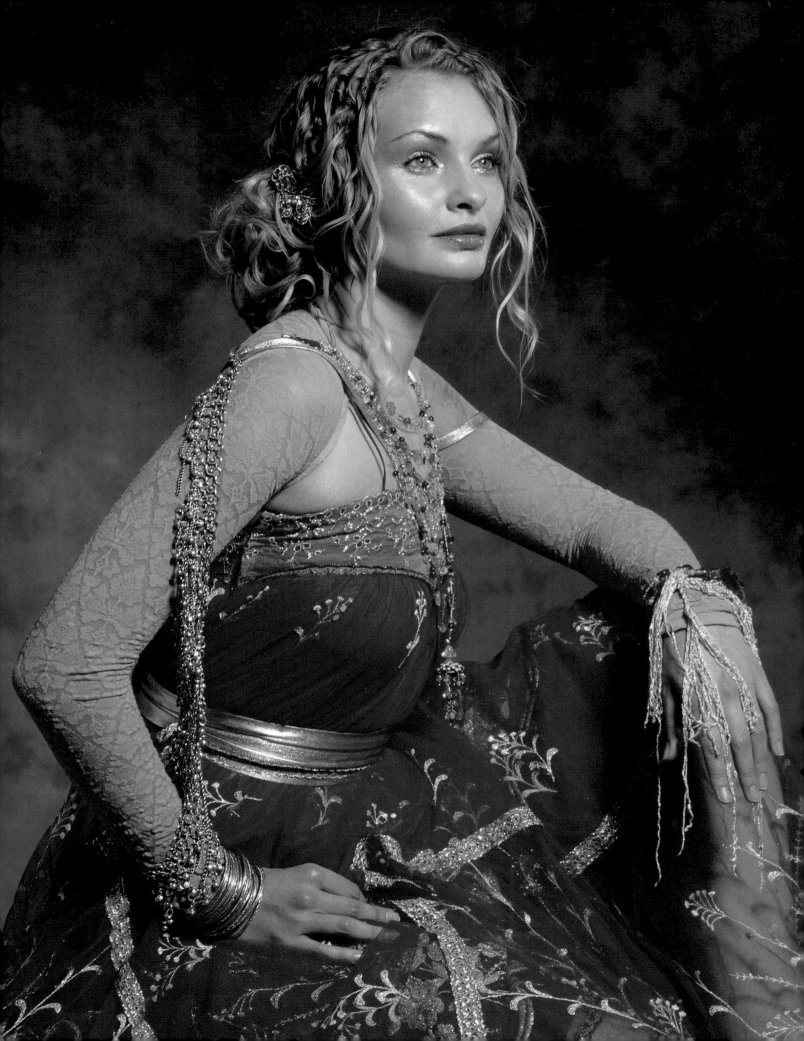

19 Twist 'n' Dry

'Utilising naturally wavy hair by twisting sections and loosely pinning the hair up at the back gives a dishevelled but romantic feel.'

TREVOR SORBIE

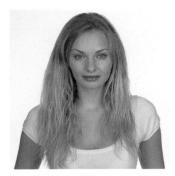

1 Before.

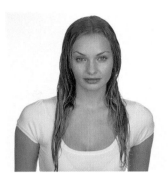

2 Mist hair with water.

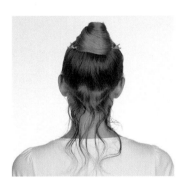

3 Section hair as shown.

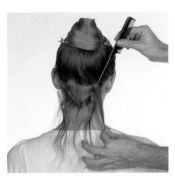

4 Divide lower hair into fine sections.

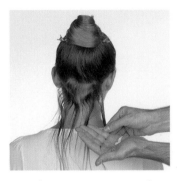

5 Work a generous amount of curl cream through lower hair from roots to ends.

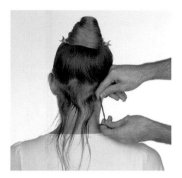

6 Twist section.

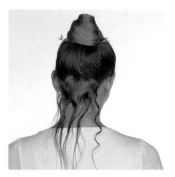

7 Shows completed first section of treated hair.

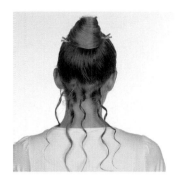

8 Work all lower hair in same way.

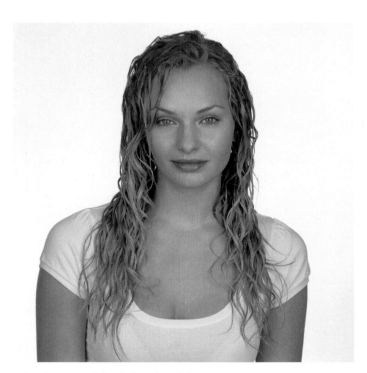

9 Let down remaining hair and work in same way until all hair is twisted.

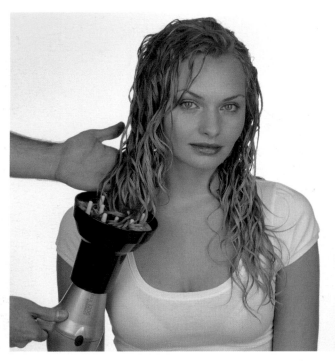

10 Using a low heat and speed setting diffuser dry the hair.

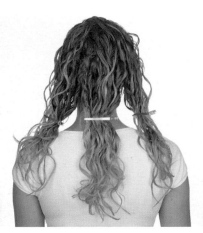

11 Divide hair into three sections and secure with section clips.

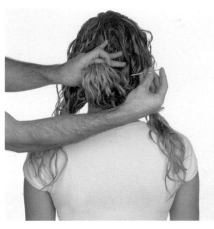

12 Roll up centre back section into a loop and secure with grips. Repeat for side sections, leaving some tendrils to fall free.

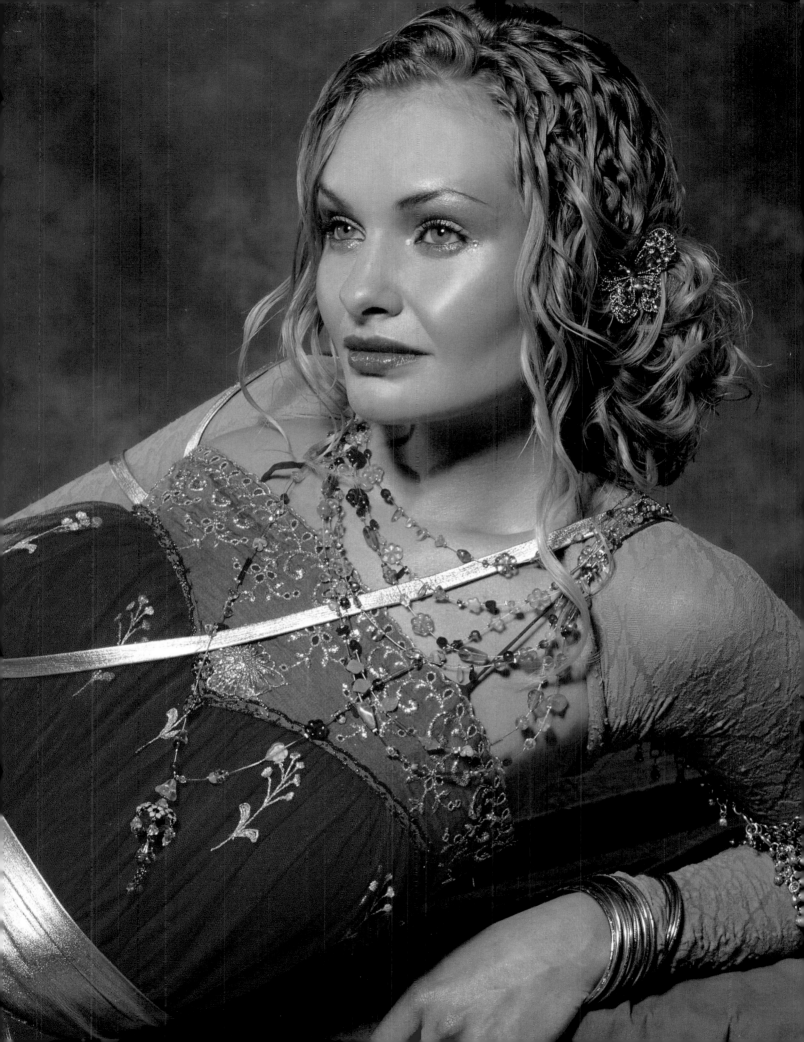

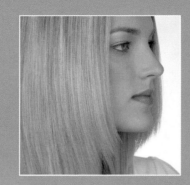

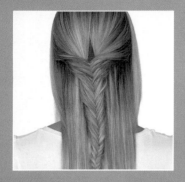

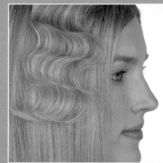

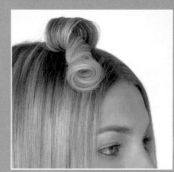

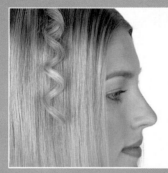

TECHNIQUES

Basic Blow Drying

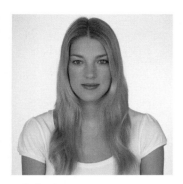

1 Before.

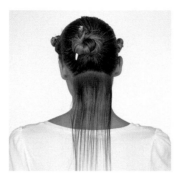

2 Section hair as shown.

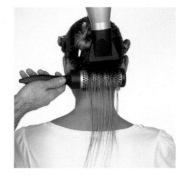

3 Begin blow drying using a ceramic round bristle brush. Use a concentrator on dryer and point airflow down the hair shaft to flatten cuticle.

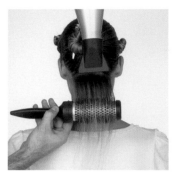

4 Continue working down hair in same way. Do not roll hair around brush, but work straight.

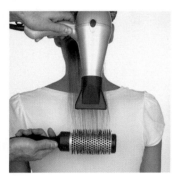

5 Continue right down to ends of hair.

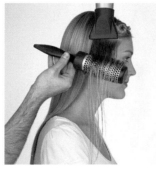

6 Blow dry rest of hair, a section at a time, in same way. Switch to cold shot at the end of drying each section to 'set' the shape.

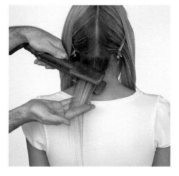

7 Part hair at centre back and, working on small sections of hair, run smoothing irons from roots to ends. Do this a couple of times before moving to next section.

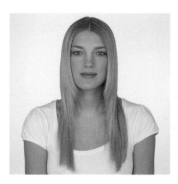

8 Finished blow dry.

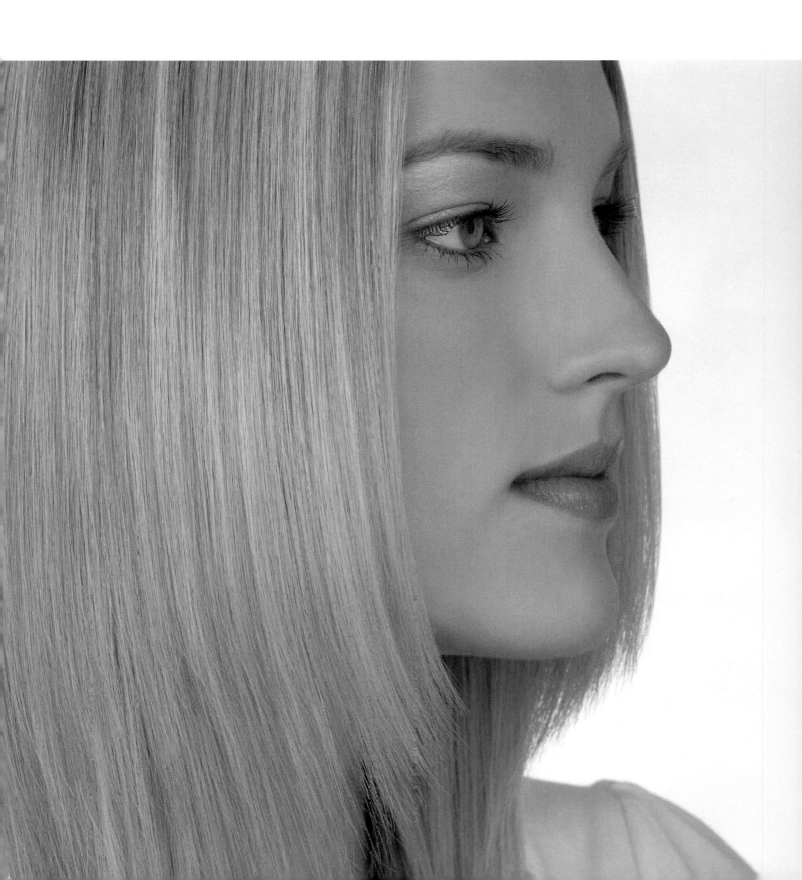

Herringbone Braid

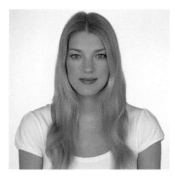

1 Before.

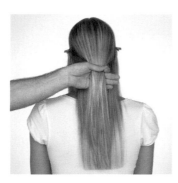

2 Section off top hair. Clip side hair to hold.

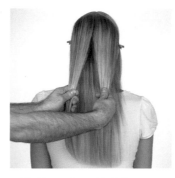

3 Divide sectioned hair into two equal strands.

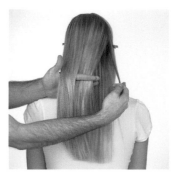

4 Take a fine section of hair from right side of the head.

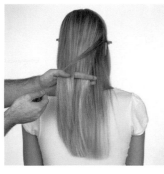

5 Move the section over your index finger and combine it with the left-hand strand between your thumb and index finger.

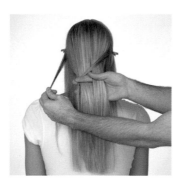

6 Transfer both strands to your right hand. Take a fine section of hair from left side of the head.

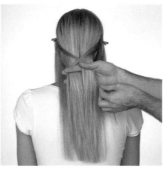

7 Move the section over your index finger and combine it with the right-hand strand between your thumb and index finger. Transfer the strands back to your left hand and repeat until there is no more hair to add. Fasten with tie.

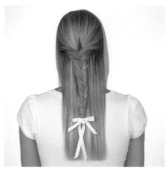

8 Finished herringbone braid.

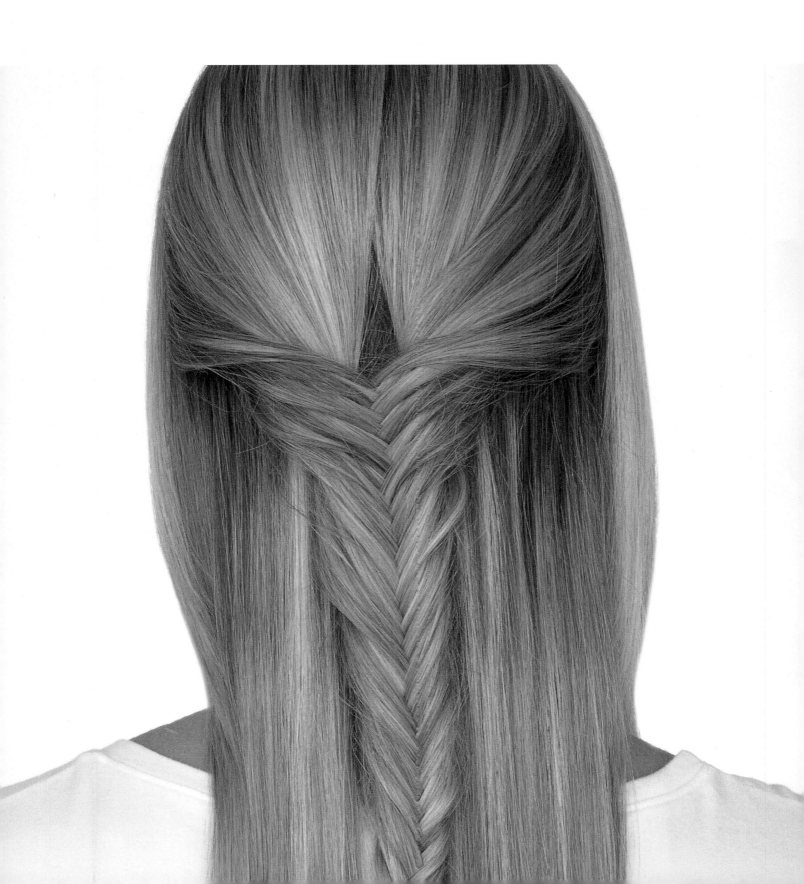

Marcel Wave

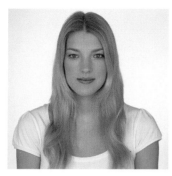

1 Before.

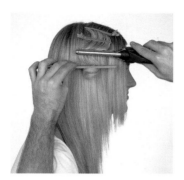

2 Take a section of hair and comb into an S shape to start direction of movement. Hold tong horizontally and insert tong and hold whilst combing next S shape of wave. Hold. Use section clips to hold waves in place.

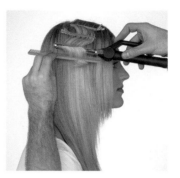

3 Tilt tong 90° whilst holding hair in place with comb to form crest of the wave.

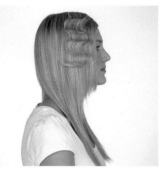

4 Shows completed Marcel wave.

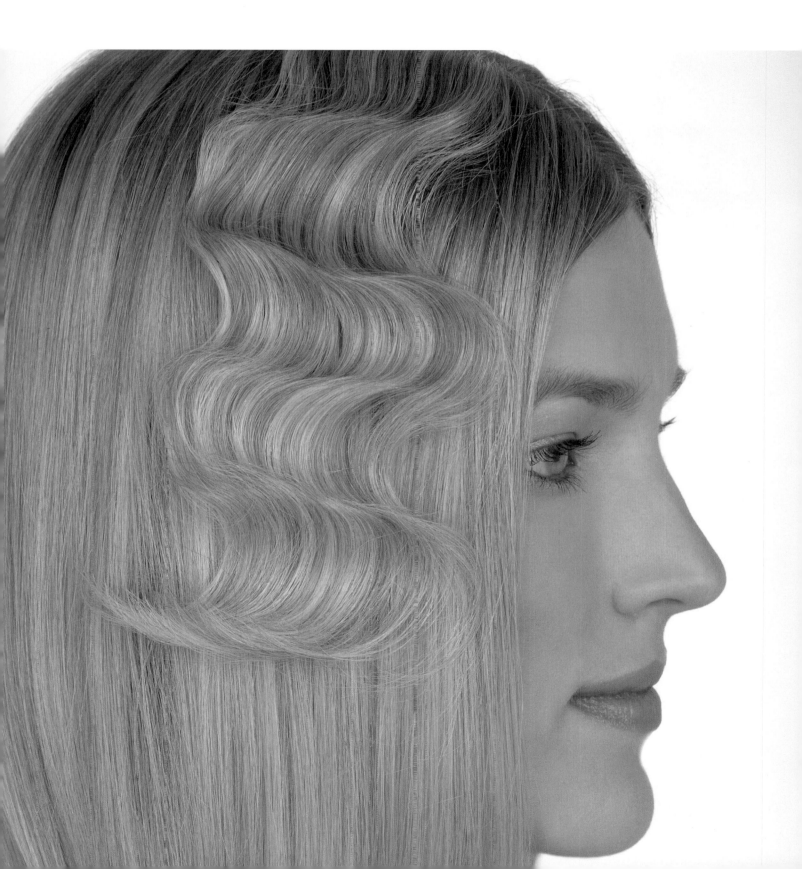

Root Curl Tonging

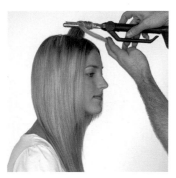

1 Before.

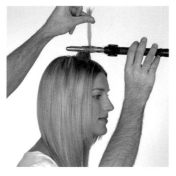

2 Take a section of hair.

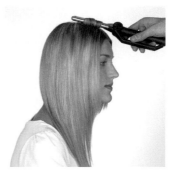

3 Insert hair between barrel of tong and hold in place with depressor.

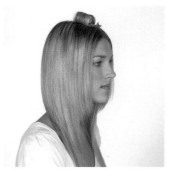

4 Wrap hair under tong and hold upwards.

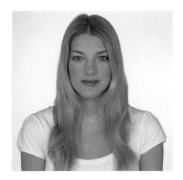

5 Open depressor and take section over barrel of tong.

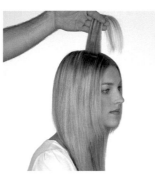

6 Twist tong in hand and bring section up as before.

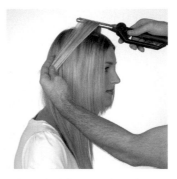

7 Repeat to end of section.

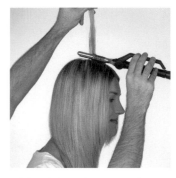

8 Shows tonged curl finished and held in place with section clip.

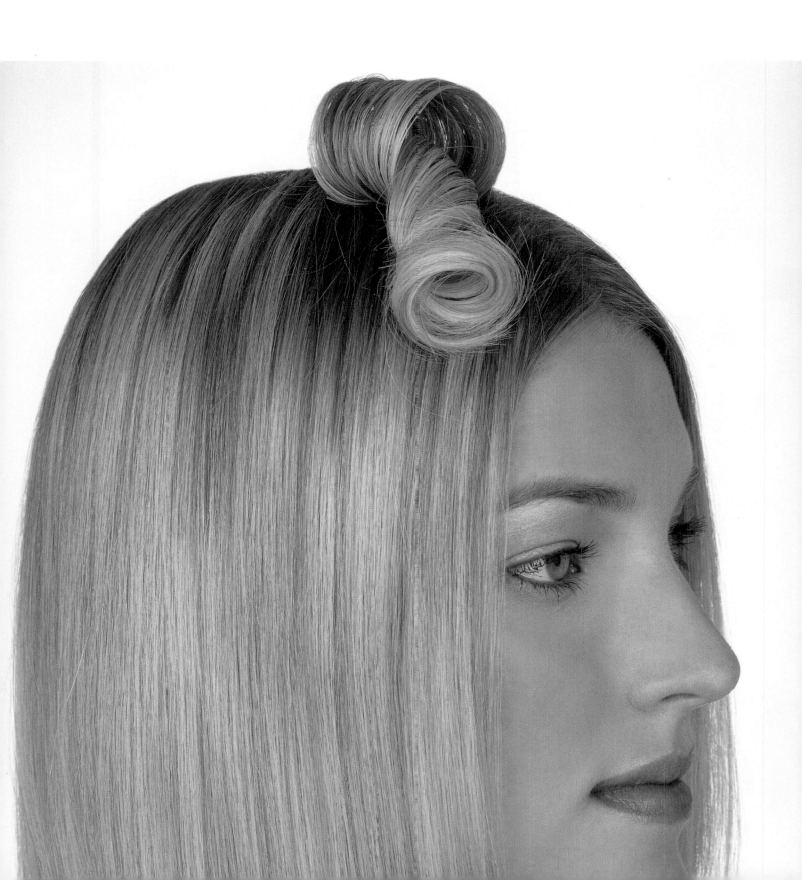

Spiral Tonging

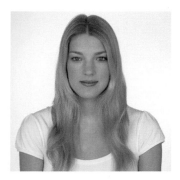

1 Before.

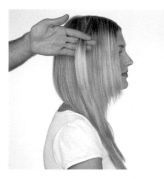

2 Take a fine section of hair.

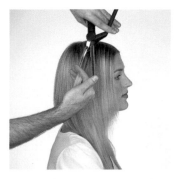

3 Open depressor on tong and insert section of hair over barrel as shown.

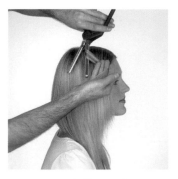

4 Continue winding section of hair down barrel of tong as shown.

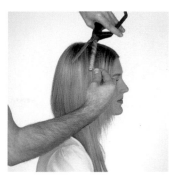

5 Wind hair right down to the end of tong, taking care not to buckle ends.

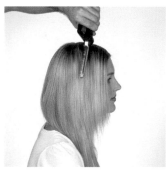

6 Close depressor and hold hair for a few seconds for heat to penetrate and form curl.

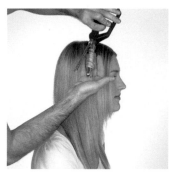

7 Release depressor and allow tonged curl to fall into your hand.

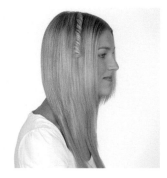

8 Finished curl, which has been released by pulling lightly with fingers.

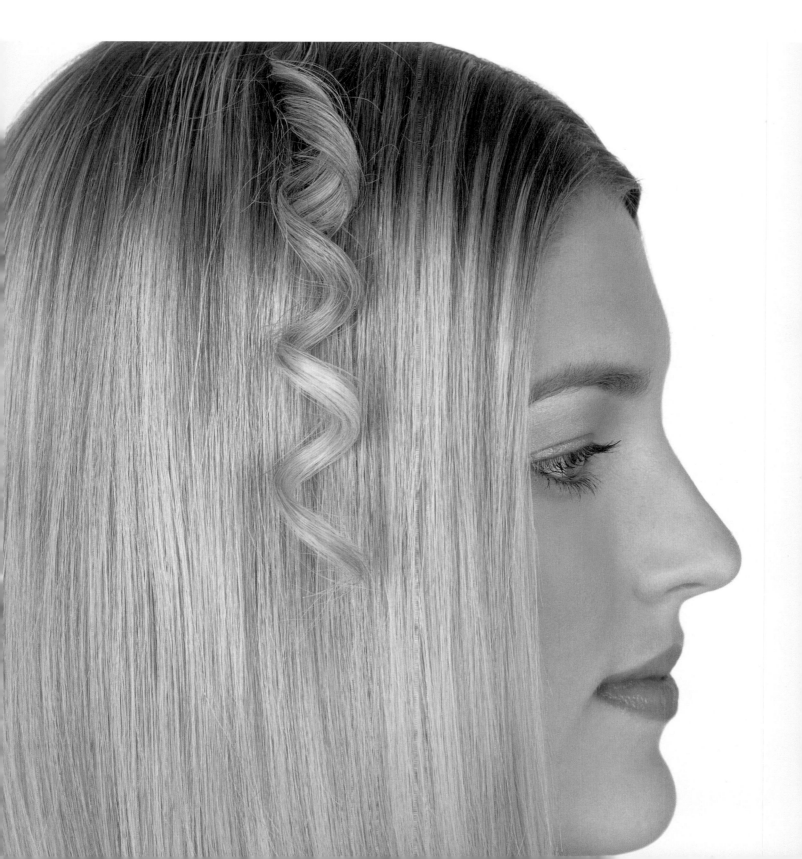

MARKETING

Reaping rewards from your bridal service

Bridal hair offers enormous benefits to your business and your self-development and creativity.

Overestimating the effort involved and undercharging are two common mistakes that leave salons uninterested in weddings. This chapter illustrates how to plan appropriately from the moment you spot that princess-cut diamond and platinum solitaire on your client's finger to the end of the big day itself.

Making the commitment

Providing a professional and confident service takes time and energy, so select one or two team members who have an enthusiasm to learn this distinctive skill; offer them formal training and the time and space to practise. Gradually add hair up and bridal hair to your in-house training programmes and let your 'occasional' hair experts share their new-found knowledge. When your client bookings hit the rainy Tuesday afternoon doldrums, encourage staff to get out their training blocks and start practising. Step-by-step books like this one should form an integral part of your in-house library and staff should be encouraged to refer to them – refreshing their memories and checking their methods should not be perceived as a weakness, rather as part of an essential learning curve. Wedding hairdressing should never be learnt on the job, so to speak; preparation and practice is the key to success.

The wedding service

'Our job is to do what the customer wants in the very best of taste', says Trevor Sorbie. A wedding is an intensely personal experience and the bride (and you) only have one shot at getting it right, so listening skills are paramount.

THE CONSULTATION

The consultation is the key part of your entire service and the very foundation for success. At this point, you will be asking many questions and helping the bride through many decisions; it is a good idea to start a file or notebook so that you can refer to it later. This will also help to reassure the bride that this element of her day will run smoothly. Invite your bridal client for a consultation at least three months before her wedding day – the questions you ask now will determine the look you create.

- *You need to know the type of dress* – is it simple or intricate? Does it have a collar or high neckline? Will the bride be changing into an evening outfit? Ask the bride to bring a picture of the dress; it may be a secret for everyone else but, like most things, she won't mind telling her hairdresser.
- *What colours are in the wedding theme?* – most brides work with a colour palette that recurs in the wedding dress, bridesmaids' dresses, flowers and reception décor. Get swatches of the colours that will be used and check that the bride's own hair colour tones well – just adding a few accents can draw the theme together.
- *What kind of headdress will be incorporated?* – headdresses are infinitely varied and can range from a few simple fresh flowers to a heavy jewelled tiara and a voluminous veil. The look you create will need to work with the chosen

headdress and if the bride plans to remove it in the evening, the style will have to work without it too.

- *Type of wedding* – is your bride choosing a traditional service? Whether your client selects the village chapel or the Little Chapel of Love, a registry office or a civil ceremony will have a big impact. Find out as much as you can about the setting and its theme, which could be ethnic, traditional, medieval so that your style will be in context.
- *The venue* – how much maintenance does your bride require? Will you be visiting the bride's home and/or the reception?
- *How tall is the groom?* – that retro bouffant might seem like a great idea now, but in the wedding photos, her man may look like a midget.
- *The Wedding Party* – do not wait until the day to squeeze in the bride's mother and the maids-of-honour. Ask if your services will be required for the rest of the party too and be prepared.

THE PLAN

The plan is the best tool you can have to keep both you and your bride on track. Based on the information you have gathered, create a detailed and timed plan that covers the following:

- *Countdown* – break your plan down into weeks that count down to the big day, so both you and the bride can see at a glance what preparation needs to take place.
- *Treatments* – salon and at-home conditioning treatments should be planned to give plenty of time to get hair in tip-top condition.
- *Colour* – make relevant colour appointments and if necessary perform a skin test.

- *Rehearsal* – book a rehearsal one to two weeks before the wedding day that includes combs, headdresses or veils. Tackle any changes or potential problems now. If you do not believe that the style is practical enough to last the whole day, then say so. Ask your bride to bring the make-up she plans to use so you can see how everything works together. Do not be afraid to suggest changes such as partings or fringes or maybe a different colour of lipstick.
- *Service times* – be clear about the amount of time your bride will have to allow on the day. Do not forget to include preparation times such as washing and blow drying.
- *Maintenance tools in advance* – give your client the products and tools she may need to help maintain her look throughout her wedding day and explain how to use them. Pressing a tail comb into her hand an hour before she walks down the aisle will do nothing for her stress level or yours.

THE WEDDING DAY

The wedding day is likely to be hectic and a little nerve wracking, so don't keep your bridal client waiting. If your client is visiting the salon, help her relax with a glass of champagne and keep her energy levels up with a few nibbles. You should be prepared, practised and have your notes or step-by-step book on hand to keep you on track and do not forget to reiterate your maintenance tips. Above all, try and enjoy the fact that you are a key contributor to someone's special day.

No price too small

Do not undersell your services. Remember that these days the average wedding costs around £15,000 and your bride will respect the service you are offering as much as she respects the florist's expertise when designing her bouquet. Under-charging is a major deterrent to entering the bridal services business, but with some logical thinking profitable pricing can be easy to achieve. Your hourly rate should be your guide and bridal hair will typically take up two to three time slots. You should remember to charge also for the rehearsal time and, if you are travelling to the clients' home, include travel costs and time. On initial consultation be clear about the amount of time involved and talk your client through the estimated costs. It is important that you introduce the Wedding Services List in addition to your regular menu and that the client understands that cut and colour are not included. Budgeting plays an important role in any wedding day, so be upfront about the total cost and clear that sneaking in the mother-in-law for a quick blow dry will add to the bill. Ask your client for a 50 per cent deposit to confirm their booking then leave all talk of money aside to focus on the real business of creating exceptional bridal hair.

Great communication

Brides have a feel good factor second to none and having one in the salon will set other clients buzzing and thinking about their own special-occasion hair needs. Wedding hair gives you the opportunity to service your client's entire lifestyle and brings you potential new business in the shape of their bridesmaids and mothers. Building your

bridal business should be seen as a long-term activity but key tools include:

- *Price list* – adding these services to your regular menu with a defined pricing structure will give them daily visibility (see opposite).
- *Portfolio* – take digital shots of your bridal clients or ask them for some shots of the big day so that you can build a portfolio to show to other clients and a notebook for yourself to record helpful hints and 'how to's'.
- *Photographs* – if you create your own hair collections, consider adding one or two dressed or bridal looks to each shoot and display them on your salon walls or in your look book.
- *Press* – wedding magazines are a genre all of their own and can always use new images. Write your pictures to CD and send them with a few words about each look.
- *Shows* – local and national wedding shows abound from early February until summer. Offer your services in the catwalk section in return for placing your salon literature on seats or in goodie bags.
- *Joint venture* – make business links with local venues, dress designers, dress agencies, jewellers, florists and photographers so that you can recommend one another.
- *Database* – include information about 'Occasional' hair in your next salon mail shot.
- *Newsletter* – write up your client's happy day in your salon newsletter and include some images from your portfolio.

Bridal Price List

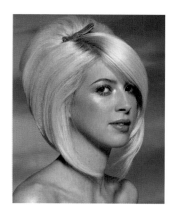

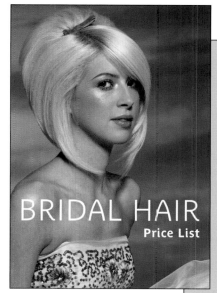

BRIDAL HAIR
Price List

Trial
IN SALON ONLY
1–1.5 hrs   Hair only £75.00
2 hrs   Hair & make-up £120.00

Wedding Day
IN SALON
2 hrs   Hair only £180.00
(min.)   plus £45 for each additional person
2.5–3 hrs   Hair & make-up £250.00
(min.)   plus £65 for each additional person
OUT OF SALON
Half day (4 hrs minimum)
             Hair only £250.00
             plus £60 for each additional person
             Hair & make-up £330.00
             plus £80 for each additional person
Full day
             Hair only £550.00
             plus £60 for each additional person
             Hair & make-up £750.00
             plus £80 for each additional person

The copyright of this photograph has been waived so, if you wish, you can download it from **www.trevorsorbie.com**. Take the image to your local print shop with typed copy of your prices and they will prepare your artwork for printing so you can have bridal price lists to give to prospective clients.

TRIAL
In Salon only

1–1.5 hrs	Hair only	£75.00
2 hrs	Hair & make-up	£120.00

WEDDING DAY
In Salon

2 hrs	Hair only	£180.00
(minimum)	plus £45 for each additional person	
2.5–3 hrs	Hair & make-up	£250.00
(minimum)	plus £65 for each additional person	

Out of Salon

Half day (4 hrs minimum)

Hair only	£250.00
plus £60 for each additional person	
Hair & make-up	£330.00
plus £80 for each additional person	

Full day

Hair only	£550.00
plus £60 for each additional person	
Hair & make-up	£750.00
plus £80 for each additional person	

Expenses are an additional charge on top of these prices and can include travel, specialist hair accessories and hairpieces.

A deposit will be taken at the time of booking (normally 50%) and added to the booking fee as a prepayment.

Clients should bring their headdress and if possible a picture of their dress with them to the trial.

Stylists will take into account the client's hair length, style or period of the dress, shape of face and height of the groom when designing the finished look.

For bookings call Trevor Sorbie

London 0870 920 1103
Brighton 0870 920 1100

Credits

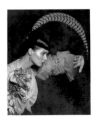

1 French Pleat MODEL: Gail

2 piece – stylist's own
Corsages and feather – Basia Zarzycka
+ 44 (0) 20 7730 1660
www.basia-zarzycka.co.uk
Earrings – River Island 0870 160 3201
www.riverisland.co.uk

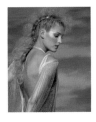

2 Fishtail MODEL: Yana

Dress – Jennifer Lang 07789 775 821
jenlang12@hotmail.com

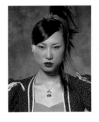

3 Top Knot MODEL: Li-Jun

Vintage gown – Rokit
+ 44 (0) 20 7267 3046 www.rokit.co.uk
Corsages – V V Rouleaux +44 (0) 20 7627 4455
www.vvrouleaux.com
Cherry necklace – stylist's own
Red polka dot bolero – stylist's own

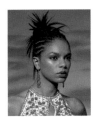

4 Rope Braid MODEL: Noella

Cream beaded gown – Rokit + 44 (0) 20 7267 3046
www.rokit.co.uk
Earrings – stylist's own
Beaded arm piece – stylist's own

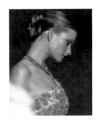

5 Twisted Ponytails MODEL: Colette

Vintage strapless beaded gown – loaned by
Andrew Fionda
Maribou wrap – Frank Usher + 44 (0) 208 551 4024
www.frankusher.co.uk
Accessories – Michal Negrin + 44 (0) 1753 861 800
www.michalnegrin.co.uk

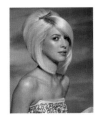

6 50s Bouffant MODEL: Jenny

1950s beaded sequin and tulle dress – Steinberg and
Tolkien + 44 (0) 20 7376 3660   www.urbanpath.com
Marcasite and cubic zirconia ring – Stockleys Jewellers
+ 44 (0) 20 7495 8066   www.stockleysjewellers.com
Ribbon – John Lewis 0845 604 9049
www.johnlewis.com

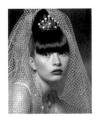

7 Audrey Hepburn MODEL: Lucie

Corset dress – Basia Zarzycka + 44 (0) 20 7730 1660
www.basia-zarzycka.co.uk
Necklace and tiara – Slim Barrett + 44 (0) 20 7352 9393
www.slimbarrett.com
Veil – stylist's own

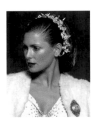

8 Short to Long MODEL: Megan

Vintage diamante studded dress and cream capelet –
Rokit + 44 (0) 20 7267 3046 www.rokit.co.uk
Brooch – Michal Negrin + 44 (0) 1753 861 800
www.michalnegrin.co.uk
Vintage rolled wax headdress – Rellik
+ 44 (0) 20 8962 0089
www.relliklondon.co.uk

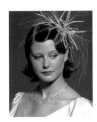

9 Finger Waves MODEL: Rosemary

Dress – Ellie & Charlotte + 44 (0) 20 8715 7150
Vintage lace blouse – Rellik + 44 (0) 20 8962 0089
www.relliklondon.co.uk
Feather/tiara – Morgan Davies + 44 (0) 20 7354 3414
www.morgandavieslondon.co.uk
Choker – Slim Barrett + 44 (0) 20 7352 9393
www.slimbarrett.com

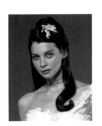

10 Top Twist MODEL: Unity

Dress – E-Racine 3 piece by Cymberline – Sarah Stalker
+ 44 (0) 7767 761 952
Choker and bracelet – Slim Barrett
+ 44 (0) 20 7352 9393 www.slimbarrett.com
Flower – AA Watkins and Watkins + 44 (0) 20 7834 8686
www.flowersforsw1.co.uk
Feather hairpiece – stylist's own

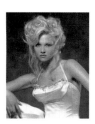

11 Bridget Bardot MODEL: Alice

Pink Duchess dress – Morgan Davis +44 (0) 20 7354
3414 www.morgandavieslondon.co.uk
Feather bag – Petals International + 44 (0) 113 266 0388
www.petals-international.co.uk
Earrings – Slim Barrett + 44 (0) 20 7352 9393 www.slim-
barrett.com
Flower – AA Watkins and Watkins + 44 (0) 20 7834 8686
www.flowersforsw1.co.uk

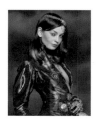

12 Coloured Wefts MODEL: Jade

Full length coat – Designed and made by Gary Page
07729 022 059
Skirt, brooches, hand and headpiece – Michal Negrin
+44 (0) 1753 861 800 www.michalnegrin.co.uk
Necklace – Slim Barrett + 44 (0) 20 7352 9393
www.slimbarrett.com
Coloured hair weft Trevor Sorbie Int.
+ 44 (0) 1372 375435 www.trevorsorbie.com

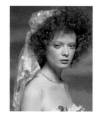

13 Frizz MODEL: Margareta

1950s Pink net tulle flower dress – Steinberg and
Tolkien + 44 (0) 20 7376 3660 www.urbanpath.com
Veil – The Collection by Ian Stuart + 44 (0) 870 600 1349
www.ianstuart-bride.com
Marcasite and cubic zirconia choker and matching
bracelet – Stockleys Jewellers + 44 (0) 20 7495 8066
www.marcasiteandmore.com

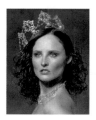

14 Twiglets MODEL: Zanne

Wedding gown – Gala – The Collection by Ian Stuart
+ 44 (0) 870 600 1349 www.ianstuart-bride.com
Tiara – Slim Barrett + 44 (0) 20 7352 9393
www.slimbarrett.com
Riding crop – stylist's own

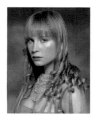

15 Spiral Curls MODEL: Holly

Dress – La petite salope + 44 (0) 20 7375 1960
www.lapetitesalope.com
Neckpiece – Slim Barrett + 44 (0) 20 7352 9393
www.slimbarrett.com

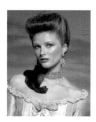

16 Scarlett O'Hara MODEL: Indre

Marriette wedding gown – The Collection by Ian Stuart
+44 (0) 870 600 1349 www.ianstuart-bride.com
Marcasite choker and chandelier earrings – Stockleys
Jewellers + 44 (0) 20 7495 8066
www.marcasiteandmore.com

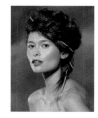

17 Dreadlocks MODEL: Patricia

Vintage gown – Rokit + 44 (0) 20 7267 3046
www.rokit.co.uk
Peach sequin wrap – stylist's own
Rings – stylist's own

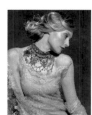

18 Coils MODEL: Rebecca

Lace dress and choker – Basia Zarzycka
+ 44 (0) 20 7730 1660 www.basia-zarzycka.co.uk
Flower – AA Watkins and Watkins
+ 44 (0) 20 7834 8686
www.flowersforsw1.com

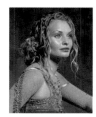

19 Twist 'n' Dry MODEL: Victoria

Dress – stylist's own
Necklace – Michal Negrin + 44 (0) 1753 861 800
www.michalnegrin.co.uk
Accessories – stylist's own

Hairdressing equipment and accessories

Sally Hair & Beauty Supplies +44 (0) 1189 443600
www.sallybeauty.com
Salons Direct + 44 (0) 151 670 9200
www.salonsdirect.com

Wigs and hairpieces

Hairaisers + 44 (0) 20 8965 2500 www.hairaisers.com
Trendco + 44 (0) 1273 774977 www.trendco.co.uk

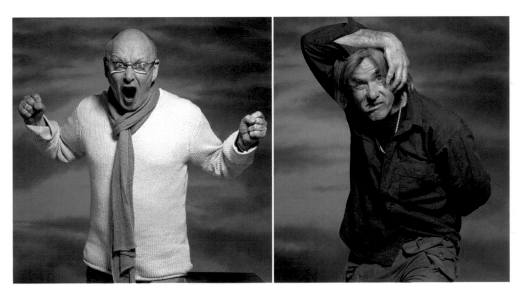

Its goodbye from Trev and goodbye from Barry (Bazza)